D1364107

THE FLYING FLYNNS

The Remarkable Adventures
of an Animal Doctor in the Wilderness

THE
FLYING
FLYNNS

The Remarkable Adventures
of an Animal Doctor
in the Wilderness

Bethine Flynn

Seaview Books
NEW YORK

Copyright © 1979 by Bethine Flynn

All rights reserved. No part of this book may be reproduced, stored in a retrieval system or transmitted in any form by an electronic, mechanical, photocopying, recording means or otherwise, without prior written permission of the author.

Manufactured in the United States of America.

FIRST EDITION

Library of Congress Cataloging in Publication Data

Flynn, Bethine.
   The flying Flynns.

   1. Flynn, Wallace J.   2. Flynn, Bethine.
3. Veterinarians—Washington (State)—Biography.
I. Title.
SF613.F58F59   636.089'092'4 [B]   79-4877
ISBN 0-87223-538-6

In memory of my husband, Dr. Wallace J. Flynn,
with all my love

BOOK
ONE

A Place
of Adventure

Chapter 1

The flickering light of lanterns fell on the figures of the men. As they went about their work, their shadows, grotesque in the dim light, flitted along the side of the barn. The whole scene was eerie, somehow unreal. I was perched on a bale of hay; an outsider, looking on.

"How would you like to go dining and dancing tonight?" Dr. Flynn had asked me earlier in the day.

Every date we'd had thus far had been thwarted by some emergency. But tonight, I thought, might be different, and I had dressed for the occasion. He, too, had dressed in his finest, and looked handsome.

We had stopped first at his hospital. "Better make sure everything's okay before we go," he said. "Want to come in with me?"

A veterinary hospital has an odor all its own, a strange mixture of animal emanations, disinfectants, and medicines. I didn't find it offensive, but tonight, as I waited for Wally to check on his patients, I was hoping my black satin skirt an lovely pink blouse wouldn't take on any of those odors.

"Everything's okay," he said as he came into the recep' room where I was waiting.

As we were going out the door, the telephone rar hesitated. I saw his indecision and hoped he wouldn't The call was from a farmer some miles north of Sea' limits, who had a sick cow.

"We'd better check," Wally said. "Won't take us long."

I had a sinking sensation in the pit of my stomach as I tried to make my voice sound casual.

"I thought yours was a small-animal practice."

"Well, mostly! I like working on large animals, but Seattle's grown so it's pushed the farmers way back. Don't get too many calls from them anymore."

My luck, I thought. One had to come tonight.

When we got to the farm, the farmer and his son, swinging lanterns, led us out to the barn. I held back when we came to the barnyard. It was mucky from recent rains and smelled strongly of cow manure—no place for a girl in spike heels.

"I'll carry you," Wally said, handing his bag to the farmer.

He picked me up as if I were no more than a sack of oats (and I probably didn't weigh much more) and deposited me on a bale of hay. It wasn't exactly the way I'd pictured myself being carried across a threshold.

The cow was bloated; even I could see that. She was stretched out on her side, her legs as stiff as sticks. Her spasmodic moos made the old barn seem even more creepy. I paid little attention to what the men were doing, but watched their phantasmal shadows grow and diminish, occasionally glancing restlessly at my watch and wondering how much longer. The minutes ticked by . . . an hour, two hours . . . and no one had so much as looked my way. Dining-and-dancing was out.

An evening in a barn was a far cry from what I'd anticipated the day I first met Dr. Wally Flynn. I'd given Maureen, my eleven-year-old daughter, a collie puppy. A puppy can't entirely replace a father who's died, but he helped fill the void. And then Laddie became sick, and we'd taken him to Dr. Flynn simply because his hospital was closest to our home.

"He has distemper," Wally diagnosed it. "He's a pretty sick puppy, but I'll do my best to make him well."

Tears Maureen struggled to control had clung to her lashes as she flung her arms around Laddie, burying her face in his coat. Wally had put a reassuring hand on her shoulder. His action somehow gave us confidence.

"You call me as many times a day as you like and I'll tell you how he's doing. Okay?"

She'd nodded and fled from the room, back out to the car.

"Please make him well, Dr. Flynn," I'd said as I followed her.

We did call him often. He didn't seem to mind. He even invited us to come and see for ourselves that Laddie was improving. But his interest in the puppy, I was beginning to suspect, had extended to include the widow. It was the way he looked at me when he thought I wasn't noticing, a sort of appraising look that I didn't discourage.

In truth, I had liked him at once, liked the crinkles around his eyes when he was amused, liked the deep, resonant quality of his voice and the dark hair waving back from a widow's peak. I even liked his mustache. And the way his muscles bulged when he lifted Laddie onto the examination table, the gentleness of his hands as he made his examination.

I liked his reaction when I told him my name. "Bethine Arndt." He'd repeated it. "Pretty name."

But most of all I liked the fact that he wasn't married. His wife, I learned, had decided not to wait when he had gone overseas during the war with a boatload of mules. Wally was thirty-nine, a good solid age, I thought, and at thirty-four I didn't consider myself too old for romance.

Romance? I shifted my position on the bale of hay for the umpteenth time and glanced again at my watch. So far, in our relationship there'd been almost everything else. It wasn't that I didn't feel concern for the animals. After all, I'd been raised on a farm in Montana. Animals in the state of Washington were certainly equally deserving. But at the moment my interest was in the man, not the animal. I sighed and turned my attention to the men.

"We've got to get her on her feet," I heard Wally say.

I watched as they fashioned a sling and slid it under her. With ropes slung over the low rafters of the barn, they heaved and tugged until they had her on her feet. And I realized, suddenly, that I was watching a man doing what he most wanted to do.

Who needed romance, I asked myself later as we sat in a roadside café savoring sandwiches and strong black coffee. I liked the man for what he was, not for what I imagined he could be.

Maureen and I had taken Laddie to Wally in early September. Our dating since had been sporadic at best. Still, I wasn't too surprised when, in late November, he asked the question I'd been waiting for. I *was* surprised, but at the way in which he asked it—by telephone, with no preliminaries, not even a "Hello."

Maureen and I needed a man in our lives, and Wally was the man I wanted. He had won Maureen over with his handling of Laddie, and he loved her. Blond, blue-eyed, a lively replica of myself, she had found her own special niche in his heart. This was important, but it had not prompted my "Yes." I loved him. It was as simple as that.

So it was that on December 25, 1948, Bethine Skaw Arndt became Mrs. Wally Flynn. It had to be December 25 he'd insisted, because "You and Maureen are all I want for Christmas."

I found adjusting to life in a veterinary hospital most difficult. I liked the arrangement of my new home. The hospital was built on an embankment that dropped off steeply. Wally's apartment and the reception and treatment rooms were at street level. The kennel rooms below, opening onto runs where the bank sloped down to a back street, were also at ground level. It was a good arrangement, but the noise and confusion set me on edge.

I complained to the kennel man one evening when Wally was out on a call. "If only I could get some sleep!"

"Why don't you take a couple of sleeping pills?" he asked.

I'd never taken sleeping pills, but why not? Lots of people did. How could I know that some people react violently to sleeping pills and that I was one of them? Stumbling blindly around the apartment, I tumbled through a window to the hard, frozen ground below, breaking my back. I had been married just over two weeks.

Fortunately for my peace of mind then, I didn't know that a friend of Wally's suggested an annulment. What damn good was a woman who would be in a cast for an indefinite time? he'd said.

"I should have mopped up the floor with him," Wally said when he told me about it later, after I, in a moment of discouragement, had suggested he might like an out. "We're in this for keeps, Chicken, so don't go getting any haywire ideas."

When, shortly after my release from the hospital, a friend suggested we go for a ride in his seaplane, Wally had strong reservations.

"In that cast? Ridiculous!"

"But I want to fly," I protested. "I can't dance. I can't play golf. We've got to have some fun. Besides, flying's in my blood. Would you believe my grandfather patented a land-sea plane? Ralph Mason Metcalf! Oh, sure, he died before he found an engine powerful enough to lift it, but it was a great idea."

Wally gave in. Somehow they managed to wedge my unwieldy plaster-cast body into the back of Al's four-person seaplane. As we sped over the waters of Lake Union and broke free, I shed my worries. It was a kind of freedom, like a gulp of clean air. I felt like a kite, soaring higher, higher! Wally turned in his seat to look back at me, raising his voice to overcome the roar of the engine.

"Okay, Chicken?"

I nodded. He shared my feelings. I saw it in the brightness of his smile.

We flew over the buildings of downtown Seattle and out over Puget Sound. I'd taken Seattle for granted before, but now I really saw it. It was a long, narrow city, bordered on the west by Puget Sound and on the east by the twenty-five-mile reach of Lake Washington. It appeared as if these two bodies of water had squeezed the land between them to form the seven hills upon which Seattle is built. To the east the foothills of fourteen-thousand-foot Mount Rainier reached out to embrace the city, and across the sound the sculptured mountains of the Olympic Peninsula held back the waters of the Pacific.

We flew north to the outskirts of Seattle to circle our own tiny claim on the city. I felt terribly proud to be a part of that white hospital and its green acre, surrounded by tall, stately poplars.

If possible, Wally's enthusiasm for flying exceeded mine. He began flying lessons that very week. The G.I. Bill would cover the cost of commercial training if he could incorporate flying into his work.

"A cinch!" he declared. "Puget Sound is littered with islands that have no veterinary service."

For a time I had to let him fly off without me, but when he obtained his private pilot's license I flew with him often. He became adept at maneuvering my rigid body into the cramped confines of a seaplane. It was glorious up there in the skies. But I wanted something more.

"It's okay for you," I complained to Wally one day when he came into the reception room, where I sat at the desk. "You have things to do."

He was silent, waiting for me to continue.

"Couldn't I help?" I pleaded.

"I'm afraid not." His answer was curt, almost a dismissal.

I caught the skepticism. How could a woman with a broken back be of any help? "But I want to help," I insisted.

Bushy eyebrows arched over quizzical hazel-brown eyes. "You are helping," he said finally.

"Yeah! Sitting in the reception room, answering the phone. Anyone can do that. I want to work with the animals."

"Oh? And do you always get what you want?"

I wasn't fooled. There was a twinkle in his eyes. "I got you," I reminded him. "Come on. You're procrastinating. You're not giving me an answer."

He shook his head, and his smile, as he leaned forward to plant a kiss on my forehead, was part amusement, part concession. He ignored a warning growl from Vicki, our little cairn terrier, who was crouched at my feet. She was his dog, but ever since I'd come home in a cast she'd assumed the role of protector. She slept at my feet at night, curled up at the foot of the bed. She refused to let anyone near me, and now, as Wally planted the kiss, she snarled and bit at the toes of his shoes.

"Vicki! Vicki!" he chided her gently. "She belongs to me, too."

He bent down to pet her, and she relented, kissing his hand, then leaping up, lapping at his cheek.

"You're a sloppy one," he told her good-naturedly, wiping his cheek with the back of his hand.

"And you're ignoring me," I reminded him again.

"Okay, Chicken!" He grinned at me, maintaining a respectful distance in deference to Vicki. "If you want to help me in surgery, I have a badly infected uterus to remove. You've watched Tom use the ether cone. You think you can handle it?"

"Of course!"

I was confident—for a time! The uterus was full of pus and blood. It was foul-smelling and nasty. Combined with the suffocating fumes of ether, it was too much. The room spun around me.

"Wally!"

Intent on his work, he didn't even glance up. "Sit down and put your head between your knees," he said. "You'll be all right."

Tom was standing by, ready to replace me. I caught the glint of amusement in his eyes.

"Oh, no you don't, Tom," I said to myself. And suddenly I saw how humorous it was. With a cast that extended from my chin to my thighs, I couldn't even bend my head, let alone put it between my knees. My faintness vanished, and I stayed on through the surgery unaided.

Wally nodded approval when it was over. "You'll do okay, Chicken. We'll make a team yet."

I continued to assist Wally in his work, on through the summer and into the fall, and succeeded in persuading myself, if not him, that in spite of my cast, there wasn't much I couldn't do.

Before we knew it, it was Christmas, our first anniversary. Wally gave me a dozen red roses, one for each month. It had been a good year, I reflected, a year of challenges, a year of growing. And now I was out of my cast, at last free to do all that I wanted to do.

Chapter 2

That following spring we bought our own plane—a little seaplane, only 65 horsepower. Our little pigeon, we called her. My mother agreed to come over from Tacoma and stay at the hospital with Maureen so we could try out our pigeon. We chose Packwood Lake, high in the Cascade Mountains, some ninety miles southeast of Seattle. The lake, a turquoise gem sparkling in the sun, was cradled at the three-thousand-foot level, and Mount Rainier loomed like a benign sentinel over the tops of towering evergreens.

"Wally," I gasped. "It's too beautiful to be true."

He nodded, too busy with the controls to reply as we swooped in for a landing. There was a tiny lodge tucked away in among the evergreens, and a dock stretching out from the lodge. We spent the night at the lodge.

The next morning, supremely confident, we climbed back into our pigeon. We circled the lake. Wally opened the throttle and pulled back on the wheel. Nothing happened. We roared around and around the lake, churning its water. Wally's lips were tight, and his hand gripped the wheel. My own hands were clenched, and I sat tensely, waiting for the feel of the lift. The feeling didn't come.

Wally spoke at last, a kind of desperation in his voice. "I'm sorry, Chicken. Only one of us is going to fly off this lake."

I swallowed. "I know," I said. "Next time you circle past the dock, slow down and I'll jump for it."

He glanced my way to be sure I meant it. I grinned, and he grinned back. "You're tops, Chicken." The desperation had gone out of his voice.

Jumping from a moving plane is not considered to be standard procedure, but if Wally lost too much momentum, he might not get off the water even flying solo. The worst that could happen to me, I figured, would be a dunking in the lake. The forward momentum of the plane held the cabin door shut, but I pushed hard against it, holding it open with my shoulder as I stepped backward onto the top rung of the ladder and proceeded on down the remaining few rungs until both feet were planted firmly on the pontoon. Holding tight to the strut, I waited until we neared the dock. Then I jumped, making a perfect landing. Second fiddle, I reflected, first to the animals and now to a plane. Oh, well! I shrugged the thought away.

Our host at the lodge came to stand beside me. We watched as the pigeon rose from the turquoise waters and disappeared over the tops of the evergreens.

"Well, he made it! Weight in those little puddle jumpers is damn critical—not," he added, "that you're packing all that much. I've got horses staked out back of the lodge and I've got a car down in the town of Packwood. I'll see you get home."

The pigeon had made it. I felt good, and I thought that for a girl who'd ridden horseback over the prairies of Montana, the six miles to Packwood should be duck soup.

The trail down the mountainside, however, was not duck soup. The steep grade was only slightly alleviated by a series of switchbacks. The horse's body raked the evergreens on one side of the trail. On the other side the mountain simply fell away, and rocks and loose gravel rattled down into the chasm with every step. My mount walked stiff-legged, feeling his way, making certain the ground under his feet was solid. This was a far cry from the loping runs over the prairies I'd known as a girl. Worse, with every stiff-legged step my body was jerked backward, then forward again. To a back newly healed, the constant jolting was slow torture.

"Whoa! Whoa there, Red!" I pulled back on the reins.

Red was obedient. He turned his head, rolling his eyes to look back at me. They were friendly eyes that did not question my decision.

I dropped the reins and dismounted. "We'll both walk," I told him. He blew through his lips, a soft rumbling sound; then, his head nodding gently, he followed me.

My guide was waiting at the next switchback. There was no room to turn his mount so he'd started to walk back.

"What happened?" he called, seeing me on foot.

"I decided to walk."

"Walk! Good Lord! It's a heck of a ways."

"Six miles or six hundred," I vowed, "I'm walking." I explained about my back.

"The trail eases out down a couple of miles. Maybe you can ride from that point," he suggested. "We'll take it slow and easy."

It was slow. At times I had to dig in my heels. Red, following, held back when the going was especially rough, seeming to know what was right for me. We became very good friends on that hike down the mountain.

The trail finally did level out a bit. I stopped and sat on the ground for a moment. Red nibbled at the grass that edged the trail, then gave me an inquiring nudge.

"Okay, Red," I said, getting to my feet. "Shall we try it again?" I rubbed his nose, and he nuzzled me affectionately, then whinnied softly, letting me know he was ready.

When I was on his back and properly seated, he eased into a slow, comfortable gait. I was almost sorry to see the town of Packwood ahead, to part company with this beautiful horse.

It seemed a long way to Seattle by car. Wally and Maureen were waiting for me at the hospital. My mother had already departed for Tacoma. I found Wally unusually serious.

"I think my horsepower was more reliable than yours," I teased him.

"Yeah!" His grin was sheepish, but then he brightened. "Maureen and I have been talking it over. I could lose maybe thirty pounds, but that's not enough. And your scrawny hundred pounds for sure can't be pared down an ounce. If we're going to keep our promise to take veterinary medicine to the islands, we'll have to have more horsepower. Besides, I leave you alone on some lake again, Maureen's going to disown me."

I caught the wink that passed between them. I gave her a hug.

"You didn't worry?"

"No! You were lucky. Couldn't we have a horse?"

"I'm afraid not. We already have about as many animals around here as we can manage."

There would have to be a new plane. We found one, an 85-horsepower Aeronca. Our new pigeon was bright yellow with maroon trim. Wally was eager to put her to the test.

"There's a lake in British Columbia I've been hearing about, Clowholm Lake. I'll get Johnny Bender to take over here. He's a good man. Call your mother and see if she'll come again." He turned to Maureen, cupped her chin in his hand. "Think you can manage your grandmother for a few days?"

The flight north to Vancouver, British Columbia, took only an hour and a half, but clearing Canadian Customs and Immigration took longer than we'd anticipated. We flew north from Vancouver, over Georgia Strait, then east up Sechelt Inlet, a narrow inlet hemmed in on either side by mountains, shadowy now in the light that foreshadowed the night. As we left Sechelt Inlet to turn up Salmon Arm, I sucked in my breath. We appeared to be flying straight into a mountain. But as we came upon it, a narrow pass was discernible, and around the curve of the mountain Clowholm Lake stretched before us, its far shore hugging the base of snowcapped Mount Tantalus. The night had a quiet mystery to it that somehow enhanced the scene's beauty.

Other concerns occupied Wally. "There's supposed to be a lodge. Where the heck . . . ? Should be lights this time of night."

"Forget the lodge," I told him. "We're running out of lake."

Even as I spoke, he "pancaked" in. This was his expression; it meant he cut speed and let the plane settle onto the water. Our pontoons cut smoothly through the black water as he slowed, then idled the engine. The shoreline was indistinct, and we still saw no lights.

"Are you sure this is the right lake?" I asked doubtfully.

"Unless our map is haywire, it's got to be. If it isn't, we're in a hell of a predicament."

Just then, from out of the darkness, came a man's voice. "Where you all going?"

"Isn't there a lodge on this lake?" Wally countered.

"Sure is! Follow me."

He'd been rowing. Now he started his outboard and led us to a small dock, where he waited to catch our wing strut. As we jumped from the pigeon to the dock, he held out his hand.

"Al Taylor here! Wondered who was coming in this time of night. Figured if it wasn't someone who knew the place, it sure as hell had to be one damn fool."

We laughed, accepting the category to which we'd been relegated.

"Bet you're hungry," he continued. "Lavone will have heard you. She'll have supper ready."

We were hungry and enjoyed Lavone's good supper of freshly caught trout. We also learned why we'd seen no lights —they used kerosene lamps. After supper Al let us choose one of two tiny log cabins.

We lit our lamp and built a fire in the old wood stove to chase the chill from the cabin. We sat on the steps of our cabin, drinking in the fragrance of fir slabs burning in the stove and the delicate perfume of evergreens stirred by a cool night breeze. Above us a star-studded sky tucked in the lofty peaks surrounding our lake. Dreamily, Wally broke the silence, sitting up straighter, his hands clasped over a knee.

"You know something, Chicken? This is for us. Someday we'll have us a place." He paused a moment. "A man has to dream, Chicken. He has to keep reaching out. You know that song, 'Don't Fence Me In'? Well, that's me, in a sense. I have an urge to go out and conquer the world. Life with me won't be any picnic."

"No one asked for a picnic," I told him. And his arms drew me to him.

He sighed and released me. "We'll stop at Friday Harbor on our way home. It's time we kept our promise. We've a darn good plane, and you've turned out to be not too bad an assistant. I think maybe the San Juan Islands can do with some veterinary service."

And I realized then that he had been waiting patiently, never by word or sign giving any indication he was waiting, until my back was well healed and I could join him in keeping his promise. At that moment I knew that wherever his dreams led him, I would be there.

Chapter 3

We had chosen San Juan Island as the site of our initial operations. The San Juan Islands had no veterinary service and welcomed us. Only fifty-seven square miles, it had a population of fewer than three thousand people, but was still the most populous island in the group and the only one to boast a town. Friday Harbor was actually more village than town. One could easily walk from one end to the other. It had a seaplane facility and was a base from which we could work.

The San Juan group, four large islands and a number of smaller islands, lie in a cluster separated by channels. Some eighty miles north of Seattle, the islands extend from the Canadian border, along the Strait of Georgia, south to a point where Pacific waters, rushing in through the Strait of Juan de Fuca, dip south to form Puget Sound.

From the air this cluster of green islands appeared to have sprouted right from the sea. Except for a few sandy beaches and some cleared areas that were proof man could not long leave nature untouched, evergeens flourish to the waterline. Most of the clearing was on San Juan Island, a predominantly landowning community, more inclined to the raising of stock than to the planting of crops.

With the help of Bill Baker, the county extension agent, who offered us the use of both his office and his secretary, Pat Taylor, we were assured of reasonable success in our new venture. An ad in the *Friday Harbor Journal* set our plans in motion. Our clinic was launched, the response to it far exceeding our expectations. We treated cattle, sheep, and goats, as well as household pets, and the island people became not only clients but friends.

It takes a certain audacity to be a veterinarian, or to be his assistant. The hogs were my first real test. Disregarding, as best I could, their offensive odor, I prepared the syringes as Wally gave the vaccines, each time darting a glance to be sure he still had both hands. There are few animals more obstreperous than an angry hog: the open snout screaming for revenge, fearsome teeth eager to shred the intruder.

"Them hogs are killers!" There was a gleam of pride in the farmer's eyes.

I didn't doubt his word. There was a meanness in their eyes that sent a shiver down my spine. If Wally saw my fear, he chose not to comment.

"Those are some beautiful animals," he said when we had finished. By comparison with certain hogs, these were beautiful. Nevertheless, I was happy their care was a responsibility we could walk away from, leaving their proud owner to take over.

We couldn't have managed without Pat Taylor, or her car. And when we needed a room for surgery, she handed us the keys to her home, not minding the ether fumes that were left in our wake, or the disarray in her kitchen. Both dogs and cats were neutered in that kitchen. We even performed a cesarean on a collie, using an ironing board propped to the correct slant. Ten healthy, crying pups had no concern for the manner of their delivery. But Wally's mind was far afield.

"There's something about a large-animal practice," he said as we got into the car. "It's so vital. Gives a man a special feeling. If our flying's done nothing else, it's given us an opportunity to fill a real need. Well, ready to tackle the next case?"

I nodded, avoiding his eyes. How could I tell him a large-animal practice gave me a special feeling, too, one hardly akin to his? But then I pulled back my shoulders and met his glance. That feeling would come. It didn't come all at once, but the next case helped. The cow had been ailing for some time, the farmer told us.

"I can't lose her, Doc. This here cow means more to me than Sarah, my wife. Sarah understands." He gave the cow an affectionate pat on the rump. "You're gonna be all right, old girl, all right!"

The barn was old and rickety, but the farmer was meticulous in the care of his animals, and the clean smell of hay was pleasant.

"Hop in that manger there, Chicken," Wally directed. "I'll get a rope around her neck. There! Pull her head to the side. Now wrap the rope around that post. Pull it up a little. Have to get into the vein in her neck. There! That'll do it. Hang tight!"

I braced my feet against the front of the manger, all too aware of the cow's terror-filled eyes staring into mine. Oh, sure, I knew about cows. As a child I'd ducked under them, gentle creatures who tolerated such antics with no show of impatience. I'd stood beside my dad when he was milking, my mouth open for the squirt he'd aim my way, laughing when he missed and the warm milk dribbled down my chin. I'd even grabbed the tails of young steers, allowing myself to be dragged across the fields. But nothing in my experience had prepared me for this nervous wild-eyed cow.

"It's okay," I murmured, hoping the sound of my voice would quiet her. "You're not half as scared as I am."

It was the horns that made my blood run cold. Occasionally I'd seen bulls fight on the prairies. I knew what horns could do, how they could rip and tear. Wally, hemmed in between the cow and the side of the stall, would have little chance if I didn't, as he said, hang tight. I took some courage from the farmer, who kept his place at the rear, a placating hand on the rump.

"Easy does it, girl! Easy does it. Doc's gonna make you well."

The soothing tone of his voice, the touch of his hand, had their effect. Some of the wildness went out of the eyes. Wally was ready. With a pad dipped in alcohol, he cleaned the area. The needle went in. The cow quivered, then quieted. It was over so quickly. I sank back against the manger, but not until Wally was out of the stall did I release my grip on the rope.

"I'll leave you some medicine," Wally was telling the farmer. "She should be all right, but I'll check in next week to be sure. In the meantime, if she doesn't act right, give me a call in Seattle. We'll make a special trip up if necessary."

We would, I knew. An hour's flight would be a small matter if the life of one of our patients was at stake.

There was much work to be done with these animals: blood samples to be taken, tests for tuberculosis, vaccinations. Friday Harbor and the environs of San Juan Island had indeed expanded the boundaries of a city practice.

Inadvertently, we had embarked on a flying ambulance service. Smaller animals requiring extensive surgery or care were flown down to our hospital one week, back to their island home the next. The cats traveled in carriers, as they are not easily handled when frightened. The sudden takeoff, the roar of the engine, was not designed to placate the cats, who howled their displeasure, spit and hissed, and dug at the wooden slats of their carriers. Though they settled down to a degree when the plane leveled out, I was thankful there was a solid barrier between us.

The dogs we transported sat on my lap or in the baggage compartment behind me. There was no choice. The compartment wouldn't hold a carrier large enough for most dogs. On one trip down, four small dogs huddled at my feet. A tight rein on each leash restrained them from leaping onto Wally's lap, which could have spelled disaster if their leashes became entangled in the controls. No flight was without its share of pandemonium and danger.

One Thursday evening in late August we had but one passenger on the flight back, a liver-and-white springer. She didn't object when we put her in the baggage compartment, but during our takeoff climb two trembling legs encircled my neck. As the legs tightened around my neck, I felt a similar constriction around my heart. Certainly I'd never anticipated being choked in midair, and by a dog. With so little room to maneuver, I felt helpless. I turned to Wally, but the crucial takeoff climb demanded his full attention. The springer's panic had to be controlled. If she lunged forward, she could send us all to the bottom of the channel.

"What'll I do?" he asked.

"Keep flying, for heaven's sake. All I hope is this darn dog's friendly." Saliva dripped from the lolling tongue and dribbled down the back of my neck. My fingers pried gently at the legs. "Let go, girl. You've got to get used to flying." I hoped my voice was soothing. "We'll get that nasty cut on your neck fixed and you'll be coming back home."

The grip relaxed. I pushed the legs away and rubbed the cords of my neck. Releasing my seat belt and kneeling backward, I stroked the springer's head. "You're no lapdog, no siree! I know it's cramped back there, but I'm cramped, too.

"Some way to make a living!" I teased Wally. "Treating patients with overdeveloped choking instincts."

Wally only grinned. The emergency was over and we were flying straight and level. I settled back in my seat. The steady hum of the engine and the soft panting of the springer had a tranquilizing effect. I could almost forget I'd been choked. Then a moist nose poked into my ear, and I turned again to face my tormentor.

"You silly old dog," I said, putting an arm around her neck. "Why can't you settle down like the lamb we flew down last week? She sat on my lap the whole way. No fuss at all. But never mind! I love you, too." I stroked her head as I thought of the lamb. A client in Seattle had wanted a lamb. We'd arranged for the purchase with a client in Friday Harbor and had agreed to fly her down. In the few days we'd had her she'd taken over our home and captured our hearts. Maureen fed her from a bottle and played with her in our yard. She was equally at home in our kitchen, temporarily replacing Vicki in that prized spot on Wally's lap.

As I mused, the stars winked on, one by one, and the moon cut a silver swath through the velvety black waters of Puget Sound. Off in the distance the faint pink glow of city lights tinged the horizon. The springer was quiet at last. I squeezed Wally's arm, sat back in my seat, and refastened my seat belt, ready for our glide back to the air harbor. This was a good life, exciting, demanding. I liked it.

Chapter 4

Wally straightened up and surveyed the bandaged leg. "Nice job, Chicken. You held the leg in the right position, kept your hands out of my way. I guess I'm not sorry I took you on."

I grinned, then became serious. "What now? No license! No one ever seems to claim these dogs."

"I know! At least the driver of that car didn't hit and run. Burns me when they leave an animal lying in the street." He laid a gentle hand on the dog. "We'll have you tearing around here in no time, Sport. Then we'll figure what to do with you."

I sighed and shook my head. "We've five or six now we haven't traced to owners." I'd hesitated to count. "We can't keep it up."

"I suppose not."

Although he agreed, I wasn't fooled. I remembered he had once said, "No animal will ever be turned away from our door, whether there's anyone to foot the bill or not." No matter how many orphans we had, we'd somehow find room for one more.

Wally always said *we* or *us*, and insisted I do likewise. "When you answer the phone say, 'We think,' or 'We've decided.' " Though the decisions must be his, he discussed them with me, and so far as our clients were concerned, we were partners.

But Wally *was* persuasive, and in a surprising number of instances someone who'd lost an animal and thought he could never love another would discover, after a few minutes with Wally, that he'd had a change of heart. No dog or cat was given to just anyone, however. The person had to be right for the animal, which was precisely the reason the number we cared for sometimes exceeded what I felt to be a respectable number.

"Mom!" Maureen called from the head of the stairs leading down to the kennel rooms one day when Sport was frisking around. "Can Laddie and I take Sport for a run?"

"My goodness!" I said, coming to the foot of the stairs so I could see her. "Are you home from school already?"

"Sure! You guys never know what time it is. Is it okay? Can Sport go with us?"

"Do you think Laddie will like Sport?" I asked her.

"He will if I tell him to." Maureen wasn't bragging or being facetious. She and Laddie were friends, and if she accepted another companion, Laddie would also.

"What do you think, Wally?"

Wally looked up from the cat he was catheterizing. "I don't see why not," he said.

So Sport went for a run that day, and for many days, until someone came to us who needed a dog—like Sport—a mixed breed. Maureen wasn't unhappy to see him go, because she knew there'd always be others to run and romp with her and Laddie.

I was once asked if I didn't find it depressing depending on animals' miseries to make a living. I said no, because animals would always get sick or hurt and I remembered how grateful I'd been to have a place to take Laddie when he was sick.

Our office hours didn't prevent us from accepting patients after hours. Dinner was interrupted so many times by the office bell that the food would be dried out from reheating, and finally, leaving a kennel man in charge, we'd dash out to a restaurant for a meal. Appeals could come any time of the day or night. Most times they were serious. Sometimes they

were funny. We'd barely gotten to sleep one night when the
phone rang.

"What is it?" I asked Wally when he'd hung up the receiver.

"Fellow thinks his dog's dying. He's bringing him in."

I glanced at my watch—1:00 A.M.! "You'd think he'd have
noticed it earlier."

"Said he and his wife had been to a party and just got home.
The dog seemed to be okay when they went out."

They couldn't have lived too far from us. We'd barely gotten
the lights on in the office when the door swung open. They
were a young couple, and extremely agitated. The husband
cradled a terrier mix in his arms.

"He's real bad, Doc," he said.

Wally's head was tipped to the side. His eyes were indecipherable. He didn't offer to touch the dog.

"Why don't you tell us about it," he suggested.

"Well, when we got home we found him in behind the
davenport. He wouldn't move. Wouldn't even look at us. We
had to drag him out. Then he just laid there."

Wally's "Hmm!" was noncommittal. Then he asked a question that I couldn't see would have much bearing on the case.
"Is this your first dog?" They answered in unison. It was.
"How does he usually act when you come home?" Wally persisted.

"Jumps all over us. Licks our hands. Gets so excited we
can't hold him down." The young man bent his head to
bestow an affectionate glance on the dog, which had not
once stirred in his arms. "We sure don't want to lose him."

Still Wally didn't offer to examine the dog. I couldn't
understand what he was getting at.

"Do you generally get home this late?" he asked.

"Oh, no!" The young wife spoke up quickly. "We're
always home early. Tonight was special. We were celebrating
our anniversary. We've been married a year."

"That is special," Wally agreed. Did I detect a hint of a
chuckle? "Put him down. Let's see what he does."

The terrier came to life, bounding around the room, yelping his delight, leaping all over Wally and me, but completely ignoring his master and mistress.

"He's crazy," the young man blurted out. "He seems to be all right now, but why doesn't he come to us? Bunko! What's the matter with you?"

Wally's eyes twinkled. "I suspect you're being punished for staying out so late. He resented being left alone that long."

The fellow looked sheepish. "Doc, I'm sorry to have gotten you out of bed, and for no reason."

"There was a reason," Wally assured him. "These little rascals can fool you. I'm glad you came. You'd have worried all night, and we wouldn't want that, not on your anniversary."

Few of our cases were disposed of so quickly. Many, like the curious cat that tumbled from the top of the chimney down into the fireplace, required weeks of care.

Responding to a frantic call, Wally had rushed off in the car to pick up the cat. I was shocked when I saw the blackened body. Not a hair remained. She smelled of ashes, and her mews were piteous. She seemed beyond help.

"We'll try to save her," Wally said. "She belongs to an old lady living alone. She's all broken up over what happened to the cat. Blames herself. Said she seldom has a fire in the fireplace, but got a notion to burn up some old papers. Poor old soul! Must be eighty at least."

Our first concern was to keep the cat alive. When she weathered the shock and the trauma and we knew we had a fighting chance, we began to take a more personal interest in her. The treatments had to be painful, yet she never protested, never tried to claw us. She was as gentle as her mistress, who called daily to check on her pet's progress. I had never seen an animal with such a will to live or such a tolerance for pain. Our Gallant Lady, we called her, and we felt a personal glow of elation when her skin began to heal and a tawny fuzz began to show. She was with us six weeks, and we came to love her as our own. The bit of sadness that comes in giving up an animal you've come to love was more than compensated for by the joy in the eyes of that dear little mistress when she took the Gallant Lady in her arms and rubbed her cheek against the soft new coat of hair.

Cats seem to have an instinct for getting into trouble. One tipped over a can of paint thinner left in a garage and was brought in yowling with pain. Another crawled up under the hood of the family car during the night to keep warm. He was badly cut in the morning when the owner, unaware of his presence, started the car.

Then there was the cat that was chewed by a dog and ran under the house to escape. I answered the emergency call.

"Can't you coax him out?" I asked the distressed woman.

"He won't come, and I can't reach him. It's a low space. I can't squeeze myself under."

"I'll be there in a few minutes," I told her.

"Where are you going?" Wally asked me when he saw me with the carrier. He shook his head when I told him. "Better let me go. Cats can be pretty belligerent."

Wally was solid and carried a little more weight than he needed. "If that woman can't get under the house," I reminded him, "you certainly can't."

He bit at his lip. "I don't like you taking chances. If the cat won't come, let it go. We'll figure another way."

"Okay," I said. "You figure while I'm gone."

The woman stood beside me as I flattened myself on my stomach and peered under the house. All I could see was a pair of yellow eyes staring back at me. I inched under as far as I dared.

"Here, kitty!" I called softly. "Come, kitty! Nice kitty!"

This cat, however, was in no mood to be cajoled. He hissed and spat and struck out with a paw, growling a warning. I knew better than to reach out for him. In his fear he'd claw and bite, and I could end up requiring more treatment than he. I lay on my stomach, feeling the dampness of the ground where the sun never hit, wondering what sort of bugs lived there, and I talked, keeping my voice low and reassuring. Still talking, and coaxing, I wriggled backward into the light, and he followed me. I could see then that one leg was torn, yet he didn't object when I reached over and scratched his neck, then tightened my grip and, with my other hand under his body, lifted him into the carrier.

One day we were called to pick up a shepherd that had been hit by a car. His mistress stood beside him, white-faced and shaking.

"It happened so fast," she said. "He rolled over and over until he hit the curb. The car just sped off."

I saw Wally bite his lips, holding in his reaction. Instead, he bent over the shepherd, sliding his hands over the body.

"I can't be a hundred percent sure," he said to the woman, "but I'm afraid his back is broken."

"Does that mean . . . ?" She could not finish.

Wally had to be honest. "If his back is broken, it's best to put him to sleep. I'll X-ray him and call you before I do anything."

Except for his breathing, he'd shown no signs of life, but as Wally, wedged against the front seat of the car, bent to lay him on the back seat, the head jerked, the mouth opened, and sharp teeth raked Wally's nose and the corner of his mouth. I stared, disbelieving, as the blood ran down his chin and onto his shirt.

"It's my fault," he said. "I know better than to pick up an injured animal without first tying his mouth shut. I wasn't thinking."

The dog's back was broken, and he had to be put to sleep. Wally's nose and the tear at the side of his mouth had to be sutured. There were scars.

"You're letting your mustache get awfully scraggly," I reproved him a couple of weeks later. I'd rather admired that mustache, always so neat and trim.

"It's going to get a lot more scraggly," he answered cheerfully. "I've always fancied a big mustache. Now I've got an excuse to grow one. You'll still love me, I hope."

I had to laugh. "I'll love *you*, all right. I'm not so sure about the mustache."

"It's not the scar," he explained. "It's having to explain to our clients how I got it."

"And how will you explain the mustache?"

"I'll just tell them," he said, "that my wife has always yearned for a man with a full-grown mustache."

Chapter 5

When I married Wally, any thought that I'd one day be flying to Alaska to help set up a veterinary clinic would have been beyond the realm of imagination. Yet here we were, this hazy June morning, winging our way north. More amazing had been the instigator.

Responding to Wally's wish for an extended summer flight, I had suggested Petersburg, Alaska. An Alaskan flight appealed to Wally more because of the distance than because a friend of mine lived there. All that was changed, however, when Sylvie Oiness's letter arrived.

She was delighted we were coming, she wrote, and perhaps we could help them as well. Many animals in Petersburg needed medical attention.

This was all the incentive Wally needed for a succession of grandiose plans. He wrote the Territorial Veterinarian in Juneau and the Department of Health in Ketchikan to determine if towns in southeastern Alaska, other than Petersburg, might want our services. The answers were yes.

Although the Alaska trip had been my suggestion, an innate sense of caution had made me hesitant.

"It sounds tremendous, but it must be a thousand miles to Petersburg along the route we've mapped. What if people don't really want our services? We've had three letters. What does that prove?"

"We'll go and find out. And don't go sour on me all of a sudden. We've made out at Friday Harbor. Alaska won't be so different."

Wally had even involved two of his friends, Dave Samman and Claire Moyer, who decided to fly with us in Dave's plane as far as Bella Bella on the British Columbia coast, where Claire had relatives.

I glanced out the window to my right. Dave was right off our wing tip. I liked having him there. To my left I could see San Juan Island. Those beautiful people, I thought. They'd agreed to a postponement of our Friday Harbor clinics. They were as excited over our Alaskan venture as we were. Everyone had cooperated. Johnny Bender had agreed to stay on at the hospital until our return. My mother had come from Tacoma to be with Maureen. All I had to do was sit back and enjoy the trip.

At Vancouver Dave glided to a landing on the muddy Fraser River, following us in. Upon leaving Vancouver, we had both become lost in a dense, smelly smog. I glanced uneasily at Wally, not needing to be told that just the brush of Dave's wing tip against ours could spell disaster. Out over the Strait of Georgia, however, we were met by brilliant sunshine. Dave was again at our side.

The Strait of Georgia and the Johnstone Strait are hemmed in on the east by the mountainous mainland of British Columbia and on the west by the nearly three-hundred-mile stretch of Vancouver Island. In between are a myriad of mountain islands. Back and forth our planes darted. The dip of a wing was a signal that some treasure had been sighted—a hidden lake, a secluded cove, a winding inlet. Somewhere in the jumble lay Sullivan Bay, where we must stop for refueling.

We found the tiny floating facility tucked inconspicuously at the base of an island mountain, its miniature harbor protected by yet another island. A half dozen buildings, set on individual rafts, extended along a narrow boardwalk. At one end was a float designed for seaplanes, with Standard Oil tanks set strategically on an adjoining bluff. Two men, un-

mistakably father and son, met us at the float. They snugged
in our planes, and I watched, intrigued, as they hauled out the
long gas hose that extended from the tanks on the bluff and
brought it across a narrow bridge and onto the float. When
someone nudged me, I was startled.

"Oh! I was so busy watching the men, I didn't see you
coming. Didn't hear you, either."

"My running shoes don't make much noise," the woman
admitted. "I'm Myrt Collinson, the third member of the
team. Sullivan Bay is a family affair, Bruce, Rod, and me.
That's it. It will take them a while to gas both planes. Come
have coffee."

Following her along the boardwalks, I easily cleared the
small open spaces where the succession of floats did not quite
meet, but I was cautious, for the narrow walks had no railings.
One misstep and I'd be splashing in the blue water that
sparkled at my feet. A step up to a raft supporting the freight
shed enabled us to walk side by side. The rafts, interlaced
with cedar logs, rose and fell with the movement of the
tides, the swell of the sea. They swayed to the slap of the
waves stirred by the wind and the rush of water from a troller
churning up the channel.

"You should feel it in a winter storm." Myrt laughed as I
struggled to maintain my balance. "Each raft, as you can see,
is chained to another, but with plenty of give so we don't
break up when the sea's running rough. We're also chained
to those rocks on the bluff, but we're set far enough out in
deep water to accommodate the freighters. We get a lot of
freight for loggers and fishermen in the area."

As we passed the freight shed and approached Myrt's
house, a brisk breeze, blowing in from the west, dissipated the
smell of the gas pouring into our tanks, but it could not overcome the briny, iodine odor of sea life on the low tide. I
stopped to admire the orange and purple starfish clinging to
rocks along the shore, and the compassfish, their multiple
tentacles propelling them through the shallow muck. I poked
at clumps of blue-black mussels masking the log supports,

and I knelt to peek under logs to spot the sea anemones, pure white and in delicate pastels, their tendrils activated by the movement of the sea.

"What a fascinating place to live. I've never seen anything like this."

"We like it," she said, and I recognized her involvement with her special way of life.

At the house a black spaniel eased himself from the porch steps and came to nudge my legs, sniffing inquiringly. Reassured, he followed along.

We passed a combination store and post office and then came upon a smaller building peeking out from a mass of nasturtiums. Mingled with their fragrance was the persuasive aroma of coffee. I hardly needed Myrt's invitation to step inside.

"Coffee's fresh," she said. "I made it when I saw your planes circling."

The coffee shop was dominated by a large coal-oil stove, its black surface shining. The coffeepot sat to one side, where it would stay hot, yet not boil. A long counter with high stools extended across one end of the room. Myrt poured our coffee, and we slid onto the stools.

"How do you manage all this," I asked, "just the three of you . . . the store and post office, the gas and the freight, this coffee shop? I get dizzy just thinking of all the work that must be involved."

"Keeps us jumping, all right," Myrt agreed, "especially if boats and planes come in at the same time. We monitor the radio for the airlines, too, but you know, it's fun. Something always happening. New people coming in, like you. We get a fair number of private planes, sports fishermen generally, but except for a few locals and those going on up to Kitimat, women are a scarce item. Tell me about yourself."

So I told her about our hospital in Seattle, our work at Friday Harbor, and our hopes of establishing a clinic in Alaska.

"Sounds exciting. I envy you."

"Me? I've been envying you." We laughed together. "I guess we're both of us fairly content with our lot. By the way, Rod looks to be about sixteen. He must have to go to school somewhere."

"Rod? Ask him about the gulls or the eagles or where to look for cod or snapper or when the run of the different species of salmon begins. He's just at home in the bush, knows every tree, where to look for deer or bear."

She had spoken oblivious of me, and I studied her openly, liking what I saw. Her body was trim and athletic. Her short-cropped hair would give her no trouble. But it was her face that held me, tranquil, yet with determination in the tilt of the chin. Here was a woman I could relate to, a woman who enjoyed doing something unusual, a woman who relished a challenge, a woman I very much wanted for a friend. Looking up, she smiled, not bothered by my frank appraisal.

"Didn't really answer your question. He takes correspondence courses. I teach him."

"Along with everything else! I bet sometimes you even pump gas."

"How did you guess?" Our laughter blended.

The voices of the men broke up our conversation. Both planes had been refueled. Responding to Rod's suggestion, Dave and Claire, along with Wally, had agreed to tarry long enough for a quick lunch. Myrt slid off her stool to make sandwiches. I studied Bruce and Rod with renewed interest. Bruce must be six feet tall, I decided, a good inch taller than Wally. Rod was a gangling counterpart of his father, but with a more animated face. A handsome family, the Collinsons!

Skippy, the spaniel, had been dozing, but now he rose, stretched, and ambled over to Wally. A few sniffs satisfied him. He yawned and lay down at Wally's feet, then sat up abruptly, pawing his ear.

"Does he do that often?" Wally asked.

"He does," Bruce answered. "So do the cats."

"Hmm! Ear mites, I suspect. I'll give you something to relieve it for now, and on our way back we'll clean those ears out—the cats', too, if you can round them up."

For Wally, I knew, the trip had now begun in earnest. He'd found his first patients. To him it didn't matter that he had no license to practice medicine in British Columbia and that his services here must be gratis. And somehow it didn't matter to me, either. After all, what good was knowledge if you didn't put it to use? I could think of no better place to make a start than here at Sullivan Bay.

Rod had been gobbling a sandwich, but left it and dashed out to refuel a newly arrived troller. Then the hum of a plane sent Bruce racing along the boardwalk. Dave and Claire followed Bruce, but at a more leisurely pace. Myrt put on a pot of fresh coffee and left, too. Rod had poked his head in the door to say she was needed in the store.

Wally shook his head. "What a place! I like it. We'd better get a move on, though. Dave and Claire will be itching to get on up to Bella Bella."

They would be for certain. For them, Bella Bella, a hundred miles on up the coast, spelled the end of the journey.

As we passed the house I heard Myrt on the radiophone, giving details of the weather. Wally didn't forget Skippy or the cats, rummaging through our bags until he found what he wanted. He handed the packet to Rod, who was standing ready to release the pigeon and head her into the wind. As the engine roared I saw Myrt sprinting up the swaying walk as easily as if it were a solid sidewalk.

"See you on the way back," I shouted, cupping my hands to my mouth. In all probability the wind carried my words away, but she nodded and waved.

Chapter 6

North of Sullivan Bay the troubled waters of Queen Charlotte
Sound battered the mainland. We chose an inland route over
Drury Inlet. Bella Bella actually was two villages, divided by
a channel of the sea. On the outermost island a Provincial
hospital dwarfed the frame houses of the Indian villagers.
Across the channel a dozen houses sprawled along the shore,
the homes of British Columbia Packer employees. They
serviced the boats of the fishermen and managed the store on
the dock where the freighters came in. The Packers, big ships
with powdered ice in their holds, carried salmon, purchased
from the fishermen, to canneries spaced at intervals along the
coast. At the far end of the docks we found what we were looking for: one float, reserved for seaplanes.

Our planes landed simultaneously, but Dave taxied in
ahead. Claire slipped a rope over the front pontoon cleat,
snubbed their plane to the float, and ran to assist us. Two boys,
about eight and ten years of age, regarded us curiously.

"Hi, fellas! I bet you're Charlie Hogan's boys."

They nodded, their eyes wide.

"I'm Claire. Your mom and dad must have told you I was
coming. How about showing us where you live?"

Still no words, but as Claire bent to pick up a bag, one of
the boys found his voice. "Could we carry them?"

"Sure! Sure you can."

Grins eased the sober expressions. Each swinging a bag, they raced along the dock to the boardwalk. Though this boardwalk was stationary—its underpinnings anchored in rocks along the shore—there were open stretches of water beneath it. Charlie's house was last in line.

He and Ann welcomed us as though we all belonged. Charlie's Irish-Indian ancestry showed in his handsome features. Nothing distressed him, not the shrill voices of the children, nor the clatter of a broken dish. He restored order without ever raising his voice.

At length Wally became serious, insisting we should be pushing on to Prince Rupert. Dave objected, reminding him he'd promised to stick around for some fishing.

"Don't worry about where you can stay," Charlie reassured us. "I won't ask you to shove in with my kids, but did you notice that big white house on the hill back of the store? Irene Tite runs a boardinghouse for B.C. Packer officials. She always has room."

"Stay as long as you like," Irene urged when we inquired. "George is on Fisheries patrol. He's gone a lot. Company officials don't come in too often. I'm glad to have company."

Wally went to get our bags, and I sank into an overstuffed chair in Irene's big homey kitchen. Then I slipped off my sandals, wiggled my toes luxuriously, and flung my legs over the arm of the chair. Wally, coming in a few minutes later, shook his head in mock disapproval.

"I see she's moved in. Can't say I blame her," he added. "Isn't that apple pie I smell? You may be hard put to get rid of us."

George came in time for supper. Later I helped Irene with the dishes while he and Wally studied their maps. The soft rumble of their voices went on and on. Irene and I paid little attention until, much later, she happened to glance at the clock.

"My goodness, look at the time! We must get to bed."

George dropped the map he was holding and jumped to his

feet. Wally and I merely looked bewildered. Not that we minded going to bed, but why so abruptly?

"The lights go out at eleven," Irene explained.

She went on to say that the village light plant was operated by an astute old gentleman who had come to the island some twenty years previous. In a sense, this was his village, and he exercised a unique control. Not only did the lights go on at his discretion, but in the evening there would be a flicker of the lights as a signal to all of a five-minute interval, then total darkness, when the village was blacked out for the night.

"I'll give you a flashlight in case you need to get up during the night," she finished.

Early the next morning we set out exploring with Dave and Claire. Channels of the sea wound deep into the mountains, dividing them into a bewildering maze of islands. Our seaplane was an open sesame to an enchanted land of sparkling lakes, tumbling waterfalls, and sheer rock walls, all framed by the intense green of the forest.

We flew and fished until the sun's golden descent sent us scurrying back to Bella Bella. There, gathered around the table at Charlie and Ann's, we recounted the day's happenings. Suddenly the lights flickered.

"We'll never make it," I groaned.

"Sure you will." Charlie thrust a flashlight into Wally's hand.

We grabbed our jackets and ran. From many windows a mellow glow offered encouragement, but only a few steps thereafter every window was blackened. We stumbled, unsure, the pallid beam of the flashlight giving little reassurance. In daylight we had ignored the possible dangers, but now, shuffling along that narrow walk, we were acutely aware of the rocks and of the sea swishing beneath us. With no railing to cling to, maintaining my balance was hopeless.

"I can't do it," I wailed.

"Shh! Everybody's in bed. Just hang on to my jacket."

"No! I'll trip over you."

"Oh, for the love of Pete!"

"I don't care!" Defiantly I dropped to my hands and knees, proceeding in this undignified but safer position.

Wally patted me on the rear. "It's gonna be a long crawl, baby."

It was, and I made certain, on succeeding nights, that it didn't happen again.

On the morning of the fifth day we were awakened by the clattering of raindrops on our aluminum roof. Music, if one would but listen, droning over and over that blissful command, "Stay in bed, stay in bed, stay . . ."

We complied, snuggling under the covers, accepting the dictates of the weather, until the heady aroma of coffee reminded us our stomachs were empty. Pushing aside our blankets, we stood shivering in front of our window, looking out on a world with so flawless a blending of sky and sea it was as if the sea had swallowed the sky, leaving our village to wallow in the mists. A gray world, but far from depressing as we clattered down the stairs, following the scent of the coffee.

The kitchen was the center of bustling activity from which emanated fascinating sounds: the tinkle of silver, the sizzle of bacon, the frantic perking of the coffee, all against a background of voices blaring from the radio. Like Myrt, Irene monitored for the airlines.

Somewhere in that encompasing grayness were planes and people. I thrilled to the part our kitchen played in the drama as the voices of the pilots filled the room, giving position reports. Staring out at the mists, we wondered how a plane could slip through. They flew as we did, VFR (visual flight rules), by the seat of their pants. As we watched, the sea and sky parted and the drone of a low-flying plane filled the kitchen. A second plane sneaked through the fog, and yet another. Their passengers filled our boardinghouse.

The pilots accepted this layover philosophically. Not so their passengers! They were strangers to the coast, lured west by the assurance of work at the aluminum project at Kitimat, a wilderness city in the making.

"What's there to do here?" groaned one. "No pub, no movie, and if I go for a walk I'll fall off that damn boardwalk and break my fool neck."

He was drowned out by voices on the radio. "Bella Bella! Your weather?"

"One moment," replied one of the pilots. Striding to the door, he flung it open. Back at the radio, his solemn report belied the laughter in his eyes. "Bella Bella . . . ceiling thirty-six inches . . . visibility twelve yards . . . winds calm, sea invisible."

"Bella Bella! Repeat, please!" a startled voice demanded.

As we listened to our report passing on down the line, nothing could have enticed me from that kitchen where our voices mingled with the unknown voices out of the air.

Then came a conversation between Sandspit radio on the Queen Charlotte Islands and an American pilot flying wheels.

"I think I'm a little off course," came his worried voice.

"Can you describe your position?" asked the Sandspit operator.

"I'm over water, but there's mountains all around."

"Off course!" snorted one of our pilots. "He's damn well lost! What's a wheel plane doing out in this muck?"

"I'm about out of gas," came the voice again. "There's a small grassy area directly below me. I'm going to crash in."

"Son of a gun!" our pilot fumed. "He ought to break his fool neck, but he just might make it. Only one grassy spot I know of, Lizette Lake at the head of Mathieson Channel."

The second pilot nodded agreement. "We'll have a look in the morning if the weather breaks."

There was no more talk of the downed pilot. How casually they had dismissed him, was my first thought. Then I realized it would be wrong to dwell on the dangers that faced us all when we flew the coast. I, too, tried to dismiss my concern for him, and succeeded to a degree. I even laughed with Wally when the lights flickered off, bringing howls of protest from the newcomers. Though they had been warned, they were not prepared. There were grumblings and muttered oaths when the guests stumbled into obstacles.

When the house was quiet and Wally lay sleeping beside me, I could not stop thinking of that crashed pilot. I stirred restlessly beside Wally. How could he sleep so peacefully? I tried again to shut out thoughts that could only distress me. But as I stared, wide-eyed, into the blackness of our room, the clatter of the rain on the roof became a sizzle on the fabric wings of our plane and I relived an evening we'd been caught in a storm. The wind had churned the river beneath us, and the night had come on with a suddenness as startling as when the old gentleman pulled the switch on the light plant here at Bella Bella.

I felt again the terror that had gripped me as Wally switched to the spare tank, that awful moment before the engine caught, snatching us from the reaching arms of evergreens we could not see but knew were there. For a time I'd wanted never to fly again. Would that pilot at Lizette Lake want to fly again? Was he even alive?

At this moment I hated Wally. I pushed away the arm that encircled me and slid to the edge of the bed. How could he drag me up this treacherous coast?

During the night the mists swirled away, and in the morning our guests were herded back to their planes. Wally and Dave, with remarkable restraint, agreed not to fly. Too many planes in that tight little area could result only in dangerous confusion. So we sat, our ears glued to the radio. At last word arrived:

"He's here! The plane's totaled, but he's okay. We're taking him to Kitimat."

Wally jumped to his feet. "Want to have a look?"

"Lucked out!" Wally exclaimed as we flew over the site. "His life wouldn't have been worth a plugged nickel if he'd hit any other spot. Why a man would fly wheels up this coast I can't figure."

Nor could I, and I frowned as we circled, the four hundred miles from Bella Bella to Prince Rupert looming, in my mind, like four thousand. And the best our pigeon could give us was eighty-five miles per hour. Flying a small plane to Alaska, I was beginning to realize, was a lot different from jetting from Seattle to New York. I could feel Wally's eyes, probing.

"You're not thinking of turning tail?"

"No," I answered.

As we flew out again, my confidence returned, and when Wally said we should be moving on, I was ready.

"I warned you you'd have trouble getting rid of us," he told Irene. "Now! There's a little matter of board and room."

She hesitated. "Would twenty dollars be too much?"

"Twenty dollars! We've been here eight days."

"I know. It's been fun. I couldn't accept any more."

Wally flushed like a schoolboy. "Well, don't just stand there," he said to me. "Say something to her."

So I did. I gave her a hug and I said, "Thank you."

Along our route to Prince Rupert there were only three settlements: Klemtu, a fishing village; Buttedale, a salmon cannery; and Hartley Bay, an Indian village. Flying the guarded channels, Finlayson, Graham Reach, Grenville, we felt only elation. Though off our route, the distant smoke from Port Essington marked our return to civilization. To the north and west of Port Essington lay Kaien Island, mainly a large mountain. On a narrow strip of land bordering the ocean roughly eight thousand people were crowded together in Prince Rupert, British Columbia's northernmost city. A quiet nook held five or six seaplanes pulled up at a ramp. We swooped down to join them.

"Welcome to Seal Cove," said the tall, thin man who caught our wing tip. "Is this a gas stop or are you staying around a spell? Name's Harold Kellough."

"Wally Flynn! My wife, Bethine! We'll stay till morning. I want my engine checked before we head up to Ketchikan. Can you recommend someone?"

"You're looking at him."

"Good enough! Any suggestions where we might stay to-night?"

"Yep! The Prince Rupert Hotel, but first I'll take you to the house to meet the wife and kids. Viv will cook you up a real feed."

"She doesn't know us," I protested.

"So? She likes company."

She did. They didn't seem too curious about our plans, but we discussed them eventually.

"What takes you to Alaska?" Harold asked. "Fishing?"

Wally's explanation surprised him. "You a doc? I'll be damned! Never would have guessed."

When Viv called us to supper, no one needed a second invitation. We lingered and we talked and the hours passed. Harold finally delivered us at the hotel at 11:00 P.M. We signed the register and were given the key to a room on the fifth floor, which was the top floor. The hotel was the tallest building in town, Harold had bragged. At the elevator we pushed the bell for service, but no elevator appeared. We pushed the bell again. Still no response! Somewhat belatedly, the night clerk glanced up from his newspaper to announce that elevator service was discontinued at 11:00 P.M.

"Wouldn't you know," I said as we picked up our bags and started up the stairs. "In this country everything stops at eleven."

Chapter 7

At last we were nearing our destination. Flying time to Ketchikan was only one hour. We were flying up Chatham Sound. Off to our right we could see the Portland Canal, the boundary between British Columbia and Alaska. Alaska! From high up in the pigeon it seemed but a continuation of British Columbia, but my heart thumped so wildly I could almost hear the beat.

We zoomed past the lighthouse at Tree Point, rocky and forbidding. There was no sanctuary there for any small plane. I listened, acutely aware of the hum of our engine. It was steady. I relaxed, looking ahead to Revigidello Island, where Ketchikan, like Prince Rupert, hugged the sea. Clinging stubbornly to the banks of the Tongass Narrows, the town was besieged by funneling winds that stirred up the waters and created excessive turbulence in the air.

We had been advised by the tower at Annette Island to check in at Ellis Airlines and clear with Customs and Immigration. Ellis Airlines was a busy place, with seaplanes coming and going, the most activity we'd seen since leaving Seattle.

Leaving our pigeon, we followed the one main street, which led to town. Frame houses, perched on rocky ledges, jutted out over the street. We stopped to admire sturdy log pillars, maybe forty feet tall, that supported a street that angled off into a residential area. We were fascinated by the hollow rumble as cars drove over the wooden planking, and we marveled at the ingenuity of the people who had fashioned a street where topography stated a street could not be. It must have taken great imagination to visualize a city on the rocky ridges of the Narrows.

My feet wanted to skip and dance. Only Wally's restraining hand in mine preserved any measure of dignity. We were looking for the Department of Health and Al Baker. In this town, where everyone seemed to know everyone else, his office was not hard to locate. He was quiet and reserved, but at the same time friendly, a characteristic of Alaskans, we were to discover. Al directed us to Herb Hetherington's Sporting Goods Shop. Herb, he told us, had been pinch-hitting as the local veterinarian.

We liked Herb at once, all six foot four of him. Eager and confident, he was direct:

"I was able to pick up a couple of veterinary manuals and I do what I can, but, hell, that's not good enough. How long you going to be in Ketchikan?"

"Not long, right now," Wally told him. "Bethine has friends in Petersburg. We're committed to working there first."

"Good enough! That will give me time to get things moving here, but when I send a wire, get back quick."

It was an order, but one to our liking. We were wanted. Our pigeon, on that hour-and-a-half flight to Petersburg, became a magic carpet that whisked us over the tops of the green mountains, across the blue channels of the sea, and over islands with strange, fascinating names like Etolin, Zarembo, and Mitkop. I phoned Sylvie at the dock in Petersburg, and Wilmer, her husband, came to pick us up. They'd about given up on us, he said, but he accepted Wally's explanation that we'd dallied to fish.

Petersburg was a small town, approximately the size of Friday Harbor; a town of frame houses and wooden sidewalks. The people were predominantly of Norwegian descent. Many of the men fished; the women worked in the cannery. A few people had cars, Wilmer among them, and there was a police officer who drove his car around and around the two-square-block business district. Petersburg seemed to be a law-abiding, churchgoing community. The need for a police officer puzzled me.

In the relaxed atmosphere of the Oiness home we worked out the details for our clinic.

"We'll need a room," Wally told them, "a vacant building preferably, where the noise and the odors won't distress any-one."

"How about that cleaning shop?" Sylvie suggested.

"I'll check. It might do," Wilmer agreed. "If you have anything else you want to do, Doc, it'll take a day to spread the word you're here. Our advertising is strictly word-of-mouth."

"Let's fly on up to Juneau in the morning then, Chicken. We promised Dr. Honsinger a call. This may be our only chance."

How we thrilled to that first night in Alaska. The sun sparkled on the sea in magnificent defiance of the hour. It was eleven o'clock, surely night by the clock, but we were as reluctant as the sun to admit the day was at an end.

In the morning rain, with dreary skies, the mountains had a ghostly appearance as we flew north to Juneau. Blue-green chunks of glacial ice were the only relief from the gray of sea and sky. Juneau, jammed between two towering mountains, was a phantom town in the mists.

Dr. Honsinger was happy we had come. Southeastern Alaska needed our services, he assured us. Busy with matters pertaining mostly to wildlife, he had no time for a private practice. He did, however, try to take care of the more serious problems in Juneau.

Juneau was like any state capital: The citizens moved at a fast pace. We preferred the more unhurried pace of Petersburg or Ketchikan, where the joy of living took precedence over matters of business. This was Tomorrow Land, where no one ever did anything today that could possibly be put off until tomorrow. Herb, with his eagerness to get us started working in Ketchikan, seemed a contradiction.

Wilmer was ready when we returned to Petersburg. The town had been alerted, the cleaning shop obtained. It all sounded great, but when I saw that shop, I was aghast. It was filthy. I chewed nervously at the nail of one finger, resisting the pull of Wally's eyes.

"No picnic, Chicken!"

And I recalled that night at Clowholm when we had sat on the steps of our cabin gazing up at a starry night. "No picnic," I agreed now. "Find me a broom. If we intend turning this place into a hospital, there's work to be done."

We went to work, sweeping pile after pile of dirt and debris. Through the grime on the window I caught a glimpse of a face, but when I swiped at the window with a wet cloth, the face disappeared so fast I wasn't sure I'd actually seen it. Certainly, though, that window needed cleaning. As I leaned forward to clean along the sill, I saw the body to that face, flat on its stomach, pressed up tight against the building. As I watched, the face rose a couple of inches and I caught the sideways glimmer of one eye. But the eye had also seen me. The head ducked back down, and the body wriggled backward around the end of the building and disappeared. I laughed aloud.

"What's up?" Wally asked.

"Some kid curious about what's going on, I guess."

With soap and water and cleaning rags, provided by Sylvie, we scoured and scraped and scrubbed. Our muscles ached, our hands were red, our faces flushed, but the place was finally clean. One problem remained. There was a toilet in a back room and a single faucet high on an opposite wall, but no sink. Wally wasn't stumped for long. Sorting through some junk in a corner, he found a hose and some wire. With the hose attached to the faucet, strung across the room and suspended over the toilet bowl, our drainage problem was solved.

"Let's try it out," he said. "Turn on the faucet."

As he washed his hands in the flow from the hose, I laughed, and couldn't stop.

"Silliest thing I ever saw!"

Wilmer, who had just walked in, agreed. "But it works. I got your lumber. Want to have a look before I bring it in? Got it as near your specifications as I could."

Wally was satisfied. They went to work with hammer and nails, first an examination table, then a six-foot-long trough for the spays. There would be spays, I was certain. Neutering female dogs and cats would help control the overproduction of animals in Petersburg. I covered the table and the trough with white oilcloth purchased at a nearby store, along with other necessary items: trays for our syringes and needles, a large wash basin so Wally could scrub up with hot water before surgery, and minor items such as sponges and small envelopes for dispensing medication. Sylvie loaned us a hot plate and a large kettle with a tight-fitting lid for sterilizing our instruments. It was beginning to look like a hospital, crude but serviceable.

While we worked, other faces had replaced the first one peering through the window. They were shy, especially the Indian children, ducking out of sight when we paused in our work to smile at them. Finally curiosity overcame shyness and heads bobbed up. Occasionally one would vanish, no doubt to carry childish accounts of our activities. Perhaps they'd even been posted to signal our readiness, for our patients were not long in arriving.

The pungent smell of soap and disinfectants in our freshly scrubbed quarters rapidly gave way to a mixture of odors: the foul stench of an infected ear or mouth, the repugnant odor of scabby bodies, the strong acrid smell of urine expelled by a nervous patient, the peculiar musky scent of the male cat, all forming a malodorous combination that resisted even the fumes of our ether.

For most of our patients this visit to a doctor was a first. They were timid, frightened, defensive.

"Let my wife hold him," Wally would suggest as the trembling hands of an anxious owner transferred his fears to an already apprehensive animal.

As Wally's hands slid over their bodies, searching and

probing, they sensed his authority. Wally had soothing hands. Just a touch seemed to dispel the fears.

For many of these patients, whose conditions had gone long unattended, more extensive treatment was indicated.

"Leave him with us," Wally would urge. "We'll give him a little nap. Then we won't hurt him and we can do a good job."

He avoided the use of the word *anesthesia*, aware of the fear the word could arouse. Even so, there were reactions.

"He'll be all right?" one gentle lady asked, tears in her eyes, when told her cocker had bladder stones.

"Is he all right now?" Wally challenged her.

She looked down at the floor, shook her head.

"Then trust us. He's going to feel so much better."

She hesitated but a moment. "I do trust you," she said.

As I had anticipated, we did have many spays. Nearly every family in Petersburg had one or more pets, pets that had families with disturbing regularity, and there was no one to give the newcomers to except friends and neighbors. Petersburg had reached the saturation point. So there were spays, both dogs and cats, and also many male cats to be neutered.

Many clients informed us we'd performed a real service in coming to Petersburg. They didn't like shooting stray dogs or drowning a batch of kittens, yet occasionally there'd been no choice.

It was satisfying to respond to their need, but what impressed me most in Petersburg was the children, who continued to pop up at our window. Their expressions were revealing. Sometimes their eyes were wide with wonder, and we knew the animal we were working on couldn't be theirs. But if their lips trembled and the tears seemed about to spill over, we knew the animal on the table was that child's very special pet and made every effort to reassure him—a smile, the thumb and forefinger forming an O, the mouthed words "It's okay." And bless them, they understood.

Chapter 8

In Petersburg there was no work on Sunday. We welcomed
the break, and after church we went to the Oiness home. Our
time with them had been mostly confined to planning and
setting up the clinic. Now we could take time to get ac-
quainted. With the two older children it was a simple matter.
It delighted them to have an animal doctor in their home.
But the three-year-old twins regarded Wally with suspicion,
peeking out at him from behind their mother. She tried to
shoo them away; they refused to budge, clinging to her dress.

I was puzzled, and I'm certain Wally was, too. He collected
people the way someone else might collect postage stamps. He
liked everybody. The mystery was solved when the little girl,
overcome by curiosity, ran to where he was seated. For a
moment she stood stock-still; then a little arm shot out, as if
attached to a spring, and tiny fingers stroked his mustache.

"It's hair!" Her voice was full of wonder.

Her brother had to find out for himself. Soon both youngsters were on Wally's lap, one on each knee. A once trim
mustache, now grown to extravagant proportions, was a source
of delight to two small Alaskans who had never seen anything
like it. To be honest, I'd never seen anything like it either. I'd
seen pictures of my grandfathers with similar growths, but in
my time they hadn't been in vogue. Wally, with his, was way
out.

"If a man wants to be known," he'd said to me once, "he has to be able to attract attention to himself. A mustache is as good a way as any."

Monday brought a terse wire from Herb: COME BACK!

We were hardly prepared for the extent of his preparations. The shop he'd procured, formerly a shoe shop, was clean and well lighted; it also had a sink. His ads, in the daily paper and over the radio, had brought results. The long list of appointments was impressive.

"You'll be here a week, Doc," he predicted, "maybe longer. Calls are still coming in. You can start work tomorrow. Today I'll give you a one-shot tour of the town."

We couldn't have found a more exuberant guide. His interest was as fresh as if it were he who had never seen it before. He showed us the theater, but explained it was the numerous taverns that drew the crowds. The main recreation, though, he said, was fishing.

"And you'd better plan on it, too," he added. "Lakes all over the place. You gotta fish if you're gonna be one of us."

Wally grinned. I knew it wouldn't take much persuasion to make him one of them.

Herb walked us all around the business area, only several square blocks.

"Meet the Doc. And Mrs. Doc," he'd say to townsfolk.

He stopped in the middle of the street, conversing with one driver, waving another around us. Traffic was slow. There was nowhere to drive except along the fourteen miles of road that extended north and south along the Narrows from either side of Ketchikan.

"See that bridge down near the waterfront and all those houses lining the other side of the river? This is probably the only river in the world where both the salmon and the men go up to spawn. Those houses are where the madams live." He grinned mischievously. "You cross that bridge, Doc, you better be carrying your black bag and have your wife with you or your intentions will be misconstrued. They go for pets, though. You'll get a lot of business from them."

The madams did arrive the next day. Herb pointed them out; a wink and we knew. Some of them must have been around from the town's rowdy beginnings. They seldom carried a purse, turning to the side to slip Wally's fee from the roll at the top of their hose or from their brassieres.

Within a few days we did get a call to the other side of the river. We stopped on the bridge for a moment, speculating about the houses and their occupants. The houses sat with their backs extending out over the riverbank and were pressed in, one upon another, in a sort of defiant togetherness. Glancing over the side of the bridge, I saw slips and panties floating in the water, carelessly tossed out from back windows.

We crossed on over the bridge and followed the wooden sidewalk along the front of the houses. All the doors were closed, all the windows shuttered, yet I had a sensation that there were eyes watching. The silence was so compelling I hesitated to break it, even to whisper to Wally. Wally's knock sounded shattering. We waited, but no one acknowledged our knock. As Wally took my hand and walked me back past those houses and onto the bridge, I felt relief. I hadn't been quite ready to enter one of those houses.

Herb grinned when we told him. "Just testing you is all. You went over together. They know that's the way it will be."

Requests for appointments kept coming in and the sign on Herb's shop, BACK IN AN HOUR, became frayed. He was always in and out of our clinic, introducing, advising, explaining.

"Doc's okay," he told anxious clients. "He's the best."

I wondered aloud if his customers wouldn't resent that sign on his door, but he shrugged my concern aside.

He saw to it there was a sign on our door, too. He made it himself. DOC'S GONE FISHING. COME TOMORROW.

Dropping in on one lake, then another, we became convinced that in all the world there could be no place more beautiful than Alaska. We fished, of course, in these lakes, accessible only by seaplane. Fish were plentiful, and the big ones had enough fight to make catching them the thrill that keeps men fishing. Wally wasn't greedy, and admired the strength and beauty of the fish, insisting that man shouldn't take more than he needs. So when we had enough for a meal, we quit fishing and lazed along the shore, or flew on to explore another lake.

I went along happily with all of Herb's suggestions until he took Wally shopping and Wally came back wearing a little green knit cap with a white tassel on the top. I rebelled.

"That's the silliest-looking cap I ever saw," I exploded.

"It's not!" Herb was adamant. "It goes with his mustache, and it's darn good advertising. There isn't a person in Ketchikan who doesn't recognize Doc when they see him on the street. You married a character, you know. Let him be one."

"Maybe it will blow off in the blast from the propeller," I suggested hopefully.

"I'll buy a couple more," Wally said, and he grinned. I said no more.

We half anticipated Herb's hesitant query a day or so before the homeward trek. "How about it, Doc? You're not going to knock it off with just this one trip?"

"Not on your life! We'll be back in September."

"Right on! Wire me. I'll have it set up for you."

I hadn't been consulted, yet I didn't mind. I felt Wally hadn't disregarded my feelings, he'd just known I'd go along.

And I didn't complain when we groped our way south through rain-drenched British Columbia channels, challenged by mists and shifting fog patches. We sneaked into Bella Bella at housetop level. Irene chided us for pushing the weather, but understood when I told her Maureen would be waiting for Wally at Sechelt after he left me off at Clowholm.

Absorbed in the challenge of our Alaskan venture, I hadn't realized how much I'd missed Maureen. We'd called her from Prince Rupert, and now I could hardly wait to be on our way, begrudging even our overnight stop at Bella Bella. But the stop paid off, for the next morning the sun smiled down, and my heart smiled, too.

I didn't mind lingering at Sullivan Bay. The Collinsons had

recognized our plane. All three were at the float when we pulled in.

"We've been watching for you every day this week," Myrt told us.

Skippy was there, too. He poked his head around from behind a barrel of oil and then trotted to meet us, his feathered tail waving a greeting. I stooped to pat his head, then stood to one side with Myrt, chatting about our trip while Bruce refueled another plane that had come in.

We strolled along the boardwalk, with Skippy, all unsuspecting, close at our heels. The men stopped at the porch, and Wally sat down on the steps. Skippy nuzzled his knee. Wally stroked his head and scratched his ears, and Skippy gave a soft little whine, lifting a paw to Wally's knee, the soft brown eyes looking trustingly into the eyes of the man. Rod sat next to them.

"Rod can hold him for me while I get those ears cleaned out." Wally said. "Go along with Myrt and round up the cats."

The cats weren't as easy to handle as Skippy had been, but with a few suggestions from Wally, Rod quickly mastered the technique, holding them tucked in the crook of his left arm, the front feet held securely between the fingers of his left hand, leaving the right hand free to control the head with a firm grip on the nape of the neck. Rod, I could see, would be Johnny-on-the-spot to help however often we stopped in at Sullivan Bay.

It had all taken longer than I'd anticipated, and I knew we'd be late getting into Clowholm Lake. Maureen could stay at the hotel in Sechelt, which was as far as she could go by bus, yet she'd be wondering what was keeping us. Too bad our pigeon could carry only two passengers!

The first faint stars had already put in an appearance when we taxied to a stop at Al's tiny dock. Wally left at once for Sechelt, a twenty-minute flight. The minutes ticked by and there was no sound of a plane. Twilight gave way to night, its blackness relieved only by the brilliance of the stars. Anxious and troubled, I paced the dock. Somewhere out there in the night were the two people I loved most.

Al sought to reassure me. "Doc will make it. Remember that first night you flew in here?"

I remembered, but to fly with the one you love in the dark of night is one thing. To be left alone to wait and wonder stirs undercurrents of fear.

At last our pigeon cut through the gap, the drone of its engine a roar reverberating from one side of the mountain to the other. The red and green lights gleamed, two jewels in the night, conducting an unseen ship into port. I reached for the wing strut, the door was flung open, and Maureen stepped down onto the dock.

"Mom, it was great flying. So smooth, all black and velvety."

"She'd gone to bed," Wally explained. "I thought of waiting there till morning, but then I figured you'd pace the dock all night."

Those next two days were all I could have hoped for. Clowholm Lake was still my favorite place. I loved the quiet, and its remoteness.

Maureen shared that love. "I wish we could live here."

"I know. Maybe someday."

But for the present, Seattle could not be ignored. Wally flew Maureen to Vancouver to catch a bus for home, then returned to Clowholm for me.

Chapter 9

"I must have been out of my mind!" A sudden violent lurch as the September winds pummeled the pigeon prompted my words.

"How so?" Wally was too casual.

"Agreeing to a September clinic in Ketchikan!" At the moment I was too distressed to realize I hadn't agreed, verbally, at any rate. "We've bucked weather every inch of the way. I've had it . . . up to here!"

"Oh, come now, it's not all that bad. Where's your spirit of adventure?"

"Right down at the tip of my toes. Sometimes I wonder what it would be like to live a nice, quiet, normal life."

"You wouldn't like it."

"Ha! I'll never know. Oh-hh!" I grabbed for the wheel as the pigeon flipped again.

Wally pushed my hands aside. "I've told you before . . . unless you want to fly this plane yourself, keep your hands off the wheel."

"I can't help it. They just fly out automatically."

"Then sit on them."

I did, and I brooded. Why couldn't we have been satisfied with our Friday Harbor practice? At least then, if the going was rough, it was for no more than an hour. But this . . . hour after hour . . . straining to see, straining to remain upright!

At dusk we sneaked through the fog into Sullivan Bay, following the vague outline of the land, barely fifty feet off the water. Myrt just shook her head.

"I don't know," I said to her later when we managed a few minutes alone. "I think I'm losing my cool. Wally probably wishes he'd left me behind."

"I doubt it." Myrt's voice was matter-of-fact, comforting, and in the morning I felt better, even though the fog was still with us. I wished it would hang in tight so we'd have to stay put. But not Wally! He paced the boardwalk waiting for it to lift. It never did, but a hazy glimpse of mountains to the east was enough for him to decide to push through to Bella Bella. Once we were out of Sullivan Bay, the winds took over, driving the fog away. I couldn't decide which was worse.

"You kids take it easy," Irene scolded when we got to Bella Bella, "and get back here before the twentieth. We often get a real blow about then."

If the real blow was worse than what we were experiencing now, I wanted no part of it. Nothing to do but sit on those hands. Wally offered comfort, belatedly, as we stood on the dock at Prince Rupert waiting for Harold.

"I'm sorry, Chicken. But we can't expect it to be fun all the way. Maybe tomorrow will be better."

It wasn't. Remembering that open stretch of sea at Dixon Entrance, we were tempted to wait. Then a call came from Ketchikan.

"Doc, you've got to come. My boxer's dying. There's a huge lump on his neck. He keeps choking and he can't eat."

We'd go, of course. Somehow I'd have to be courageous.

"We'll head right out," Wally was saying. "We'll use your kitchen for surgery. Have plenty of hot water and clean sheeting material ready."

How could you have been so reluctant, I chided myself later. The dog didn't even raise his head when we walked into that kitchen, but as we unpacked and sterilized our instruments, mournful eyes followed our every move. He didn't flinch as we gave the injection. With so much pain, what was one more prick? The eyes closed, and we lifted his inert body to the kitchen table, prepared with layers of newspaper and then the sheeting. Wally sterilized and draped the surgical area. His incision was quick and sure. From it poured a foul mixture of pus, blood, and serum.

"Why didn't you let me know sooner?" Wally asked the relieved owner when we had carried the boxer back to his pallet.

"I knew you were coming, Doc," the man told us. "Herb had it in the paper. I thought old Alex could hold out until you got here. Guess he almost didn't."

"You were stretching it," Wally agreed. "This has taught me a lesson, too. From now on, especially with the winter months coming up, emergency cases will have to be flown to Seattle. We can pick the animal up at the airport and keep him until he's okay."

"We'll rest a hell of a lot easier up here with that assurance." The man stooped and stroked Alex's head thoughtfully. "It's a long time till June."

"You kids ought to move up here," Herb said later. "Look at you now. You're swamped. Hardly take time to eat."

It was true. We worked far into the night. It was often 3:00 A.M. when we staggered back to our hotel room. Everyone shared the concern of the boxer's master. We shared their concern, and though we were overburdened with work in the short periods we were here, we knew the fluctuating population couldn't support a year-round veterinarian. Herb reluctantly admitted we were right. Besides, we needed the hospital in Seattle, its equipment and its facilities, to back up the work we did here.

That fact was forcefully demonstrated when a cat whose jaw had been shattered was brought in by an elderly couple.

"Poor Thomas!" the woman crooned, stroking his back. "Poor Thomas! We never should have let you out."

"Do you have any idea how it happened?" Wally asked.

She shook her head. "He's such a gentle cat. Why would anyone want to hurt him?" She looked at her husband. Numbly, he shook his head, too.

Wally didn't press for more information. "Leave him with us," he said. "We'll do all we can for him." But when they were gone he voiced his thoughts. "Can't hardly blame it on an automobile. Traffic moves too slowly, what little there is. Looks more like someone picked up a two-by-four and let him have it. Sure would like to get my hands on anyone who would pull a stunt like that."

With Thomas anesthetized, we could make a more detailed examination.

"Damn!" Wally muttered. "This is the worst mess I've seen. Sure wish I had him down at the hospital. All we can do here is wire that jaw together and hope it holds."

First the mouth had to be cleaned. Bits of bone were removed, and teeth that were hopelessly loose were taken out. It was painstaking work and could be done only little by little. Wally could work for a time, then it was up to me to swab out the saliva. It seemed impossible we could make that jaw workable again, but we were patient and persistent. When we were finished, I knew it was a job well done.

There was the danger of infection, however. "I want to see Thomas again tomorrow," he told the Clarks when they came back for him. "In fact, I want to see him every day I'm here, and when we go back to Seattle I want you to send him down to us. I should X-ray that jaw. I want to make sure those wires hold, and I'll need to keep watching for any sign of infection. This will be slow healing. He'll be with us a month, maybe longer."

"We don't mind how long you keep him, Doctor, if only he gets well," Mrs. Clark declared. "I know he's only a cat, and there's some would say he isn't worth it, but to us he is. You call us as soon as you get home. We'll send him."

By commercial airlines it would only be a matter of hours. It seemed strange, when we stopped to think of it, that people up here hadn't taken advantage of the airlines before. Was it a perversity of human nature that made them want to know the man who would doctor their pets? Herb agreed that was at least partly true.

"Before you came, Doc, people took it for granted if there

was nothing that could be done for their pet here, he'd best be done away with. A lot of dogs were shot around here— that is, unless Betty King got wind of it. Someday you might meet her. You might say she's an eccentric, but she's also a remarkable woman, and her concern for animals, believe me, is unsurpassed. She has a big old house back in the bush. Won't let anyone near the place, but rumor has it, and I believe it, that she has at least a hundred and fifty dogs back there."

"Wow! Where did she get so many?" I asked.

"Asked for them at first. Some way she'd hear the police were going to shoot a stray. She was always right there begging them to let her have the dog. Actually, no one cared much whether the dogs were shot or whether Betty had them, just as long as they weren't running the town in packs. Then it got so people who had a sick or an injured animal, or one they just plain didn't want, would be in touch with Betty."

"I'd really like to meet that woman." Wally's interest was definitely aroused.

"You won't meet her unless she wants you to," Herb advised him. "But we all know where to look for her. She makes the rounds of the cafés and meat markets, asking for scraps. Mostly you'll see her going up the alleys. Generally has some of her dogs with her, on leashes. Takes no chance of losing one. If someone wants her they leave a message at one of the cafés. She takes the animal and that's it. From then on it's hers."

"Why didn't you tell us about her when we were here in June?" Wally asked. "Maybe we could have contacted her."

"Nope! You couldn't have. Getting used to the idea of you being here will take some doing on her part. She pretty much considers Ketchikan her territory."

"You mean we're not welcome . . . as far as she's concerned?"

"Not that, exactly. It's more like she has to make up her mind it's right for you to be here."

"And she doesn't make up her mind in a hurry, I take it."

"You got it . . . as far as people are concerned. With animals . . ." He snapped his fingers. "Like that!"

"Strange!" I observed. "She didn't just happen. Does anyone know anything about her background . . . where she came from?"

"Not much. There's been talk she was a cook for some famous dancer who began collecting strays after her husband died, somewhere in the Midwest. Then she died, so the story goes, and left her money to Betty so Betty could carry on with her favorite charity. I don't think anyone really knows just when Betty showed up here. No one pays much attention. People come and go. It's kind of a restless population, really. People come in expecting to make a fortune, fail, and move on."

"I see," Wally said. "That's why there's always been a vacant shop for us when we come."

"Right! Of course, a lot move on just 'cause they can't stay put in one place. You'll find that out in your work. You may treat an animal here once, then never see it again. Oh, we have a lot of old-timers who'll never budge. Betty's one of them. She'll be here till she dies. I'd bank on it."

Chapter 10

Would the rain never stop? Even after our return from Alaska, it persisted. We were absorbed in cases that had accumulated, those who preferred to wait for *their* doctor. The realization of our inattention to practical considerations came with startling suddenness one night, jarring me out of a sound sleep. Wet, trembling with indignation, I screamed at Wally.

"How dare you pour a bucket of water over me?"

Usually hard to awaken, now he rolled over quickly and stared at me. I was too angry and confused even to wonder how he could have committed such villainy while sound asleep. His bellow of laughter infuriated me even more.

"What's so darn funny?" I demanded.

"You are. All that plaster in your hair!"

I felt my hair, looked at the bed. The rain, beating on a flat roof, had found a weak area and collected in a spot directly above my head. The ceiling literally had fallen in on me.

"Not a drop on you," I complained bitterly.

The roof was fixed, and the rain gave way to snow, so heavy that our Friday Harbor trips had to be curtailed. Even our pigeon was endangered. We didn't fully realize this until the day an urgent call came from the air harbor.

"Doc! Your plane is sinking."

The weight of the snow packed on the wings of the pigeon was slowly forcing her under. We hurried to her rescue as fast as the icy streets would permit. As I watched Wally climb up on the engine and scrape the snow from the wings, I wondered why so many unusual things kept happening to us. Were we careless, or was it just fate? Wally would say fate. "If it's supposed to happen, you can't stop it," he always maintained. I was more inclined to think that was an easy way to absolve oneself of responsibility. But at least we'd gotten to the pigeon in time.

The weather continued stormy, but our clients in Alaska didn't forget our injunction. Thomas had arrived, of course, and periodically we made other trips to the airport to pick up an animal needing attention. For a time, they, too, became members of our family.

Vicki ruled the household by right of seniority. She had been mistress long before I came to challenge her authority. She accepted each new member but tolerated no nonsense from them. Laddie had long since desisted in his efforts to get her to play. I had a kitten, a Mother's Day gift from Wally, who quickly learned Vicki was not one to tangle with. Minx was a lovely kitten, with subtle blendings of black, red, and orange. I cringed at times, fearing Vicki's methods of discipline were too severe. Still, Minx grew into a well-trained, obedient cat.

Obedient to a point, that is, for now she was pregnant, and we accorded her certain privileges warranted by the dignity of her condition. She had been my cat, purring herself to sleep in my lap, jumping to my shoulder in playful moods. Now her favorite spot was Wally's worn easy chair. No one, save Vicki, had ever dared trespass. Minx knew better than to challenge her for the warm depression left in the cushion when Wally rose to tend a patient.

"What's got into her?" I demanded. "She knows she's my cat."

"Just a whim. You know how it is when you're pregnant."

I wrinkled my nose at him. I didn't see how either of them could be comfortable, but neither budged. There Wally sat, Vicki on his lap, Minx squeezed in at his back, until the day she began squirming, pushing against him while emitting plaintive little mews. Her time had come.

Then there was another mew, shrill, demanding. A grin spread across Wally's face. He twisted in his chair, then held out to me, in his big cupped hand, a tiny moist replica of the mother.

I held out my hand for the bit of life squirming in Wally's. He pinched the cord and placed the mite in my hand.

"Get some soft toweling and rub it dry," he said.

It mewed, lifting a tiny head, shaky and unseeing. It crawled about in my hand on unsteady legs. Such a fine, healthy kitten.

Now a second mite mewed its confusion. Then a third, a fourth, and a fifth. Minx knew that was all. She jumped to the floor with remarkable agility, as if giving birth to five kittens was no chore at all. Oh, she was proud! She wanted acclaim, and demanded it, rubbing against our legs, purring in a self-satisfied way that said plainly, "See what I've done."

I dropped to my knees beside her. She responded to my voice, to the touch of my hand, arching her back as my hand passed over it. The purring increased in volume. She was my cat again.

Wally, meanwhile, had prepared a bed for her and placed the babies in it. Minx, heeding their cries, turned from me. She didn't settle down to satisfy their hunger as a normal mother should. She stood in their midst, hesitant, uncertain. Then, with one mewing mite in her mouth, she leaped into Wally's chair, depositing her infant in that still warm depression where he had been sitting. She left the kitten there, mewing lustily, while she went for the others. Vicki eyed her uncertainly, but made no move to interfere. Satisfied, Minx lay down with her family. Instinctively they searched for, and found, the source of the milk. Their hunger appeased, they slept, and Minx, her soft body curled around them, slept too.

Wally knelt beside Vicki, pulling her close to his knee. "I guess we'll have to let her have it, old girl," he said.

"You mean you're going to let Minx have your chair?" I asked.

"Of course! What kind of a heel would I be, evicting a whole family!"

And then the door swung open and Maureen sailed into the room, stopping short as her eyes fell on the kittens.

"Minx," she cried, "you've got babies! Why didn't she wait for me to come from school? I wanted to be here."

Maureen dropped to a sitting position on the floor, her chin resting on the cushion, her eyes never straying from the sleeping kittens.

Although I sympathized with her love for each of our pets, I was also irritated by what I considered an overdose. I had told her repeatedly that Laddie could not sleep on her bed. Oh, but they were the sly ones, waiting for my goodnight visit, Laddie on the rug beside the bed, Maureen snuggled down in the covers. "Night, Mother," she would murmur. Laddie would raise one lid, and I could see that "What are you going to do about it?" look in his eye. When I would tiptoe in later, I'd find him sprawled on the bed with Maureen perilously close to the edge, clinging to it with the tenaciousness of the subconscious.

I complained to Wally, who was no help. "They're happy, aren't they? If he pushes her off some night, they'll work out some other arrangement."

"I'm sure!" I replied. "Maureen will sleep on the rug and Laddie will have the whole bed. And it's not funny," I added, detecting a twinkle in his eyes.

I never quite became reconciled to their arrangement, but I couldn't stay angry with Laddie. He was a lovely dog, always so content to run in our acre. Then one day he disappeared. What had enticed him, and how he'd managed to scale our eight-foot-high fence, we couldn't know when we found him lying in the street. He was alive when Wally lifted him and carried him to the hospital. Maureen followed quietly, her hand gripping mine.

When Wally examined him, his voice was grim. "I can't save him."

Harsh words! To Maureen he had been more than a man, more than a father. Now he was failing her. I couldn't accept it.

"Why?" I cried. "There's not a mark on his body."

"Internal injuries. The wheel of the car must have gone right over him." With thumb and forefinger he held the eye open. "See the whiteness." Gentle fingers parted the passive jaws. "Look at the gums . . . no color. He's lost blood, too much."

Maureen's sobs tore at my heart. "Can't you do something?"

"I'd do anything, but . . ." He turned to her, a sense of inadequacy clouding his eyes. She went to him, still sobbing.

"I'm sorry, honey." His voice shook as the big hand patted her shoulder, and I saw his pain, too. It was Laddie who had brought us all together. "There's life and there's death," he went on. "In our time we have to experience both. Sometimes it's rough."

Time and again that night, when I tiptoed to the door of her room, I could hear anguished sobs, muffled in the covers.

"Leave her be," he said. "She's got to let it out."

The sobbing continued, the next day and the next. She stayed in her room, avoiding our sympathy. When, obediently, she came to meals, she merely toyed with her food. My heart ached at the sight of her red and swollen eyes. School was out of the question.

"I can't stand it, Wally. I don't ever want her to have another dog."

"That's no way to talk, Chicken. Of course she'll have another dog. This is rough medicine, but if she doesn't learn to accept it now, grief could overwhelm her in later years."

The crying did stop, but the tired eyes and the droop at the corners of her mouth tormented me. How could one compensate for so great a loss? Wally suggested she look at a puppy he had downstairs, but she shook her head. He didn't push it, but a day or so later he approached her again.

"Come with me, Kitten. I want to show you something."

She hesitated, knowing what he wanted to show her, not wanting to see it, but she went. I followed. We stopped before a kennel where a small black-and-white puppy stood with her black nose poking through the aluminum bars. At sight of us the whole body wriggled, then whipped around, and she leaped against the kennel door. "Take me out!" It was a demand accentuated by shrill yips.

Wally put an arm around Maureen. "No one wants her," he said. "You have so much love to give, and so many puppies need someone to love them. Don't you think you could take one?"

Still hesitant, she opened the kennel door. The puppy leaped into her arms, yelping with delight, covering her face and neck with moist kisses. She looked up from the squirming puppy, and I saw a glow in her eyes, a tiny smile easing the droop of her mouth.

"I'm going to call her Spif, 'cause she's, well, she's just spiffy." And she snuggled her cheek against the baby-soft coat.

Spif was an unruly bundle of energy, positive everyone wanted to play. Vicki growled low in her throat when the teasing became too bothersome. Minx swatted her meaningfully to show her annoyance, but the kittens loved her. Her long tail, waving like a plume, was irresistible. She would slide across the kitchen linoleum, five kittens in hot pursuit. When she skidded to a stop, they were all over her. She rolled and kicked and bit at them. They kicked and bit back, but it was all in fun. No bite ever broke the skin. When Maureen joined in the ruckus, they climbed over her, swatting her playfully. Now her eyes sparkled and her laugh was for real.

Spif was still very much a puppy when Gardenia joined our family group. A client brought her in.

"Can't keep her any longer," he explained. "I took her home when I accidentally ran over her mother, but she's a smelly little rascal. Sprays at the bat of an eye. My wife gave me an ultimatum. The skunk went or she would. Hate to turn the little pest loose. We've gotten her so domesticated I'm afraid she can't fend for herself."

"I could de-scent her for you," Wally suggested.

"No! Sorry! My wife wouldn't have her if she smelled like a rose. She's a cussed little creature. Do what you like with her."

"Couldn't we keep her?" Maureen pleaded.

"I don't know, Kitten. We have quite a houseful already."

He couldn't resist the plea in Maureen's eyes. Our newest member had to be de-scented, for it was plain she didn't intend to be cooperative. The show of white teeth and the shrill screams were not signs of affection, but a chunk of cotton, saturated with ether and dropped into her box, took the fight out of her. When she became groggy I applied the ether cone, and Wally removed the objectionable scent gland.

"What will you call her? I asked Maureen.

"Gardenia!" she answered promptly.

Gardenia never even knew what had happened to her. In fact, she was so sure her defense mechanism was functioning that whenever she was irritated, which was often, she would go through the entire procedure, stamping her feet, then turning swiftly and lifting her tail, positive she had given us the works. We all felt her ire, but overall she was lovable, and at times even loving. She liked sitting in our laps, especially if the lap was already occupied. Using her long, curved black nails and her strong white teeth, she climbed easily, though the furniture suffered. Nudging, shoving, she would dislodge whatever occupant the lap held and then settle down happily. Only Vicki refused to be budged. They would push back and forth, neither giving an inch, finally settling down together with a mutual respect.

She was an obstinate, contrary creature, impervious to scoldings. Her favorite tidbits were walnut meats and cheese, and she soon learned where each was kept. She knew which she wanted at any given time. Standing on her hind legs, she would take the hem of my dress in her teeth and tug, pulling me to her objective.

"Doggone it, Gardenia," I scolded one day, "you're tearing my dress. I've had enough. You're going into your kennel."

I picked her up, forced her teeth apart to free my dress, and plopped her into her kennel. She stomped and lifted her tail, giving out with that peculiar scream that told me she was angry indeed.

It was a mistake. She had been unresisting at bedtime. After a session on whichever lap suited her fancy at the moment, it had been a simple matter to pick her up and carry her out to her kennel. But this evening, when Maureen slid a hand under her body she slithered to the floor and, with a speed remarkable for such short legs, darted for the living room and scooted behind the davenport. I knelt at one end, Maureen at the other. Beady eyes glared at me, and somehow, in those confined quarters, she managed to twist her body around so her back was to me. Then she lifted her tail.

I clapped my hands, and she ran toward Maureen. "We've got you, you rascal!"

"No we haven't, Mom. I couldn't hang on. She's too wiggly."

She *was* too wiggly, I realized as we chased her round and round the furniture. Several times we had her cornered, only to have her slither from our grasp, screaming as she did so. She was positively infuriating. On her next round she stood up by the coffee table, pulled several magazines to the floor, darted to the desk, tipped over the wastebasket, and stomped through the spilled contents.

Wally had been checking a patient, but at that moment he opened the door and stood there surveying the mess.

"What in the name of . . . ! What's going on in here?"

"Gardenia won't go to bed," I snapped with clenched teeth.

"Let her be. She's still a wild animal. You should know better than to try to pick her up against her will."

"I should have known better than to agree to keep her in the first place. I'm sorry, Maureen, but honestly, it's like living in a madhouse."

"Oh, come now!" Wally had gone to stand beside Maureen.

He put an arm around her shoulder, and I knew that against the two of them I didn't stand a chance. He sided with her, but it was me he spoke to. "Have a cup of coffee and cool off."

"What about Gardenia?"

"Forget her. She'll settle down once you quit chasing her. Maybe she has other ideas about where she wants to sleep."

I sat down with a cup of coffee, and Gardenia, satisfied the chase was over, waddled back to the kitchen. I swore I detected a look of triumph in those calculating eyes as she surveyed the room and its occupants. Vicki, disdainful of all such nonsense, was asleep on her pallet. Minx was curled up with her kittens, content to leave well enough alone. Maureen's hand was on Spif. Spif would have delighted in joining in the ruckus, but she had learned fast that Gardenia was not one to be tampered with.

It had happened at feeding time. Vicki always sat up, waiting sedately for the command to eat. I had taught Minx to follow Vicki's example, and the kittens learned from her. Spif and Gardenia had been more difficult to persuade. Now all would sit on their haunches, their forepaws fanning the air until the signal was given. Their manners left much to be desired. Only Vicki and Minx showed any restraint. The kittens pawed through each other's bowls and edged in beside Minx until she said, "That's enough," and swatted them.

Spif and Gardenia slurped their food, ever hopeful of barging in on someone else. Their methods differed, however. Spif would merely nose her victim aside, snatching up the last morsel of food. Gardenia would waddle to the bowl of her choice and cover it with her broad black-and-white tail. Woe to the one who tried to trespass. Spif, tail wagging, had tried it, just once. Quick as a flash Gardenia had a foot on that tail, and then, deliberately, she bit it. I recalled Spif's surprised yelp as she pulled away.

Gardenia, head up, little black nose sniffing, was making her decision now. Whose bed would she take? It didn't take her long to decide. Nails clicking against the floor in emphasis, she waddled straight to Vicki and climbed up beside her.

"What does she think she's doing?" I was still unforgiving. "There's no room for her with Vicki."

"What do you want to bet she makes room?" Wally asked. She did. Squatting and shoving, she inched Vicki over. Vicki grunted, not even bothering to open an eye, but there was room for two now if close proximity was agreeable to both. With Gardenia's luxuriant tail spread over Vicki like a coverlet, the two of them settled down to sleep.

Wally grinned and winked at Maureen. "Well, that's settled."

Chapter 11

"Too tired for a snack?" Wally asked, holding out my jacket.

"Not if we can find a place that is open."

"The hotel café's open till midnight. I checked."

We turned the key in the lock of our temporary veterinary clinic and stepped out into the night. Our street was deserted, but as we rounded the corner, the blare of a jukebox punctured the night and loud voices and raucous laughter exploded through the open door of a tavern. One fellow, braced against the building, regarded us through bleary eyes. A not-so-young couple, holding hands and snickering over some inanity, brushed by him as they entered the door.

"What a town! But you know something . . . I love it."

"No place like Ketchikan," Wally agreed as we approached the café.

The café was almost deserted, but the waitress bustled over to our booth as if she were pressed for time. We studied the menu she gave us and decided on breakfast, ham and hash browns, since we probably wouldn't have time in the morning.

"Nice indigestible bedtime snack," Wally observed.

Our day had begun with a little old lady who came in with her Snooky. She was terribly embarrassed to have to tell us that such a ladylike dog would go out in the yard and eat her own bowel matter, but felt better when Wally told her it was a condition that could be corrected, just the dog's system demanding certain minerals.

"It always surprises me a little," Wally said, "how willing people are to cooperate here, like the fellow who brought in Rowdy, for instance. I'm glad I was able to persuade him to leave him. That anal gland was badly infected."

The waitress arrived with our "breakfast," and we attacked our food with gusto, neglecting talk. Then Wally's thoughts intruded, and he paused, fork in midair.

"You know, it was worth the whole trip just to be able to help that old cocker."

I knew the one he meant and shuddered, remembering how those nails, every one, had grown around and back through the pads, some of them even working their way through a second time.

"Damndest thing!" Wally continued. "No wonder the poor dog had trouble walking. First time I've had to use an anesthetic to cut toenails."

"You'd think they would have noticed. Arthritis, they said. Imagine!"

"Could seem like arthritis if you didn't look. I'm not too surprised they didn't notice those nails. That long hair that grows between the toes of some cockers hides a multitude of sins. I hope we can persuade people to keep that hair cut back so they can spot trouble before it gets beyond control. Looks prettier long, they say." He shrugged, then laid down his fork. "If you've finished, Chicken, let's hit the sack. We've a heavy schedule tomorrow."

I nodded. No matter how carefully we parceled out our time, we always seemed to be running behind schedule. There were always emergencies or someone in from out of town who hadn't been able to make an appointment. I was ready for bed. Morning would come soon enough.

We started that morning with surgery, three dogs and a cat to be spayed. Then Wally had several consultations, and I ran back to the hotel to check on calls. As I pushed open the heavy doors, the desk clerk addressed me.

"Hello, Mrs. Doc. There's a call for you."

I liked the "Mrs. Doc." It meant I wasn't merely the slave who wiped up urine, sterilized the examination table, and scrubbed instruments. Not that these duties were omitted, for they are an integral part of any clinical setup, but my work—assisting in surgery, instructing clients in home care—gave me a special feeling.

Now I was puzzled. The clerk had addressed me without ever looking up.

"How did you know who I was?"

"Hell, Mrs. Doc, the minute you opened that door I smelled you." My eyes widened and my mouth dropped open, but he seemed not to notice. "That ether you're wafting is mighty potent."

"I didn't realize the odor clung to my clothes that much."

"No apologies! Folks up here don't mind how you smell. We're darn glad to have you. Here's your number."

I made the call and hurried back to the clinic. Wally looked up as I entered. "Anything urgent?"

"One call. I gave him an appointment for tomorrow."

"Good, 'cause we've got our work cut out for us for this afternoon." He pushed open the door to a back room. "Look what we've got."

"Doberman pups! Five of them! I didn't think they had any Dobermans in Ketchikan."

"They don't, as far as I know. These came in on a troller from some little town about seventy miles from here."

"Beautiful pups! Wants their ears cropped, I'll bet."

"Yeah, and the works—distemper shots, complete checkups —and we've got to get moving. The fellow who owns them wants to get started back as soon as possible. Better get to sterilizing right away."

Ear cropping is an exacting art. It is no simple matter to crop ears so they will stand erect, especially if there is a weakness in the ear structure. Often they require manipulation after surgery. Wally studied these ears thoughtfully.

"I believe they'll stand," he said. "They've got to. We won't be seeing them again."

They did stand. They were beautiful. Wally was pleased, and so was their owner when he came for them.

"I heard you was good, Doc," he said. "These ears prove it."

Later in the day Al Baker stopped in to see us. I smiled as we shook hands, remembering that day, our first trip to Ketchikan, when we had walked into his office wondering how to get veterinary medicine started in Alaska.

"I came in for an appointment, Doc," he said, and at Wally's look of surprise, "Yep! Fran and I talked it over and decided on a cocker pup. She's three months old, but what we don't know about a dog would fill a book. It's up to you, Doc."

Wally paused a moment, checking our appointment schedule. "Is ten o'clock tonight too late for you?"

"Make it later than that if it fits in better with your schedule."

"No. Ten will be fine."

Brownie's checkup that evening was purely routine. We gave her a distemper shot, checked her ears, her eyes, her teeth, checked for worms. Through it all she remained happy, her moist tongue caressing our hands, her back end waggling.

"Fine animal, Al," Wally concluded with a final pat on Brownie's head. "You'll love her."

Al nodded. "We do."

Herb was in and out these days in his customary breezy manner, organizing our calls, advising, threatening if he felt we were overdoing it.

"You kids knock it off," he insisted one afternoon. "You haven't even had lunch. I know. I checked at the café before I came. And stop by the desk. There's a call for you."

We had a quick lunch, then picked up our call. Wally rang the number, and I stood leaning against the wall, only half listening. A mounting flush on Wally's cheeks drew my attention. In our work, dealing with all manner of people and all types of conditions, many most intimate, he was not one to be flustered.

"I'm sorry," he was saying, "but we've had to make it a rule not to make house calls. We just haven't the time."

There was a pause while he listened to the voice on the phone. Then: "Yes, I understand. Yes, of course. Just a moment, please." He clamped his hand over the mouthpiece and turned to me. "It's the madam. You know the one, the recluse. Her cat has a badly infected ear, she says."

"Well, why doesn't she bring it in?"

"She says she has seven cats and she's not going to drag them all down here. I about told her to go to hell, but then she said weren't her cats as deserving as anyone else's. Put me on the spot, dammit!"

"Okay! Let's go. Herb will sit in at the clinic till we get back."

He grinned sheepishly. "She said, 'Don't bring your wife.' "

I giggled. "So that's what all the confusion is about. Tell her you'll come."

"I could tell her I won't come without you."

"And make a client unhappy? Go along."

He told her he'd come. Then we went back to the clinic to collect the medicines he'd need. Herb howled when we told him of the condition she had set.

"Doc," he said when he could get his breath, wiping tears of laughter from his eyes, "you'll never live this down. She's the queen bee in this man's town, that's for sure, even if she does live way out by herself. She's just selective about whom she sees is all."

Wally wasn't gone long, but it was apparent he'd been impressed. He described in detail the scrolled gate to the grounds, the winding, evergreen-lined road leading to the mansion, the maid who let him in, prim and rather severe, and the mansion, plush, but all in good taste. He paused, wondering how much he should tell us.

"Come on! Give!" Herb prodded him.

He grinned and shook his head as if still finding it hard to believe what he'd seen. "*She* was something else," he said finally. "When she came . . . well, dammit! She sort of floated in on a cloud of perfume, wearing a long white satin gown that flowed around her. Dynamite! She isn't young, but she gives an impression of agelessness. Her face is remarkably unlined, and her hair, a sort of blue-gray, was piled high in a bun, I guess you call it. Anyway, she was unreal. It was like looking at a picture, even to the jewels. Man! Earrings, bracelets, a necklace, and a ring on every finger, and believe me, those jewels weren't junk."

"She sounds like a production," I observed, "but how did she come by so much money?"

"Not too hard to come by in Alaska," Herb assured us. "Men get lonesome. They'll dump all their earnings in the lap of anyone they favor."

I shrugged, accepting his explanation. Then I asked Wally, "How about the cats? Did you get around to them?"

"Damn right! They were pampered and spoiled, not in need of too much attention, but I went there to check them, and by golly, I checked them, every one."

There was one thing he hadn't told us. "What did she think of you?" I asked.

Laughter rumbled from deep in his chest. "I think . . . disappointed," he said, and we joined in his laughter.

Our next case was simple enough. It was the explaining that was difficult. This client had just come in from the back country. He had that lean, hard look that one connects with men who have lived most of their lives in the bush.

"My dog ain't ailing," he informed us, "but when I heard there was a doc around I figured I might as well bring him in. Damn good hound! Whatever you say he needs, I'll pay for it."

"What's his name?" I asked.

"Hound! That's what he is and that's what I call him."

Wally didn't find much wrong with Hound, but since the dog lived in the bush and had contact with wild animals, he thought it wise to give him a rabies vaccination. Then Wally suggested that a stool sample be brought in. The request for stool brought a puzzled frown.

"I ain't got no stool, Doc."

Wally hastened to explain. "I want a sample of bowel material. See! My wife's examining some now."

The man stared at the sample in the jar, from which I'd

removed a speck with a swab stick. I was in the process of smearing it on a slide for examination under the microscope.

"Hell, Doc!" His voice registered disbelief. "That's just shit! 'Pears like you got 'nough round here already, but if you want some more, I'll get it."

While I bent over the microscope, hiding my amusement, Wally attempted to explain he thought Hound might have worms, but needed to check the bowel matter to be certain. Our man was unpersuaded, but agreeable.

"Okay, if you say so. Hell of a way to make a living, though, messing with that stuff!"

Wally suggested he look through the microscope and see for himself a round egg I'd found. At first he could see nothing, complaining the aperture was too damn small.

"Take your time," Wally advised. "Your eye will adjust to it. See it now?"

"Well, damn! Yeah! I do. Pretty good, huh? Never saw in one of these damn things before."

The microscope had intrigued many of our clients. It excited them to see for themselves the ear mite, or mange mite, or worm egg. The fact the animal had parasites was of less importance. They expected the animal to have some problem. They expected us to correct it.

But when Tina, the ten-year-old dachshund, walked in, I knew this was a case that would not have a happy ending. Her mistress had left her with us so we could make a more thorough examination. Her enlarged mammary glands were raw and bleeding, for with every labored step she took, they scraped the floor.

"Poor old thing! Is there any chance we can help her?"

"I don't know." Wally ran his fingers through his hair in a gesture of helplessness. "Those enlarged glands in themselves shouldn't cause all the symptoms we're seeing. She's too emaciated and too listless. I'm sure there's malignancy. I should persuade Mrs. Bean to let us put her to sleep."

This was a difficult decision, not only because of the sorrow inflicted on the owner, but also because the doctor must acknowledge to himself that medicine has its limitations. Yet it wouldn't be right to let this animal suffer longer or to give her mistress false hopes. There were tears, of course, but Mrs. Bean accepted our prognosis.

Fortunately, in most of our cases we could offer a happier solution. I was glad we could help the shaky little orphan fawn Al Baker brought in. Someone had found her alongside the road and brought her to Al.

"Can't get her to eat a darn thing, Doc. Won't even take milk, and she has diarrhea something fierce. If we can't stop it, I'm afraid we'll lose her."

Weak as she was, she resisted our efforts to give her the necessary medicine. Finally Wally squirted it into her mouth with an eyedropper. Then he gently rubbed her mouth until she salivated and was forced to swallow. I got her to eat by dipping my fingers in milk and forcing them into her mouth. She soon sucked on them willingly, and it wasn't many days before she was taking food on her own. When she was eating well and running about, Al turned her out in the woods in back of his house, where she could roam at will, but still seek out human companionship as long as she desired it.

Our routine was interrupted one afternoon when a man burst into our clinic, staggering under the weight of the golden retriever held in his arms. The dog was snorting and slobbering and in evident distress.

"You gotta do something, Doc," the man said. "He's got a fishhook caught in his mouth. He's the best damn bird dog in the country. I got a camp up island. Get a lot of hunters. I can't lose this dog."

We gave the dog an anesthetic and put a clamp in his mouth. The hook was caught at the base of the tongue. It was delicate work. We did not want to injure the tissue.

"Gad, Doc!" the owner exclaimed when we had finished. "I'm glad as hell you were around, but you sure as hell don't charge enough. Twelve fifty! That's nothing. I'd pay any amount and figure I got off damn cheap." With that, he shoved a bill in the pocket of my uniform.

Such a thing had never happened to me before. I stammered a refusal, but he brushed my words aside.

"Keep it, dammit! Do you know how grateful I am?" And I saw there were tears in the eyes of this rugged individualist. I knew that not only did he need the dog, he loved him as well.

I thought of the many wonderful people we had met up here, and I regretted that many of them we might never see again, like the genial owner of Monsieur, a standard French poodle. He and Monsieur would be trying their luck farther north, he'd told us.

"Mon Sewer!" he threatened now as the dog sniffed the table leg with its tantalizing odor of urine. "You lift your leg and I'll kill you." Then he turned to us, pride in every fiber of his voice. "Damn smart dog! Understands every word I say."

There were those, however, we could depend on seeing each time we came. For cats, Jean Backshas had a heart as big as all outdoors, and for her cats she wanted the best. There were always nails to clip, ears to clean, vaccines to give, as well as a number of spays and castrations. During our absences she'd lose some, to disease or through some accident, but she always adopted others, so that she generally had about a dozen. Some of the strays she took in infected the others with ear mites or worms or maybe mange, but this never deterred her.

"I know you folks can take care of it," she said.

People like Jean, like Herb, were Ketchikan to us. So was Mary Hirabayshi, with her short black hair and her happy face. She had a little café near the waterfront where she featured both Japanese and American dishes, and she, too, collected cats.

"Ketchikan would not be such a good place if we did not have cats," she explained. "Otherwise too many rats."

Although she needed the cats to keep the rats from infesting her place of business, she, like Jean, loved them and felt an obligation to take care of them. She also had a dog, a husky named Curly. Curly was an obstinate creature, who didn't take to all the care and attention Mary felt was his due. I think he never really liked anyone except Mary and her son, Gilbert. After a number of visits, having been told repeatedly by Mary that we were his friends, he did accept us without baring his teeth and curling his lips. We felt we'd made real progress. Despite the husky's image as the Alaskan dog, Curly was the only one in Ketchikan.

Mary was someone special to us. Sometimes, late at night, when we were walking back to the hotel after a long day at the clinic, our route would take us past Mary's café. It would be dark, even upstairs, where she lived. Then a window would open and a voice would call down to us.

"Mrs. Flynn! Mrs. Flynn! Would you like a cup of tea?"

In a moment the lights would flash on downstairs. We'd hear the grating of the key in the lock, and the door would swing open, revealing Mary, smiling and bowing and urging us to come in. From somewhere she'd produce a couple of pillows, which she plumped down on the benches on either side of the table. We never had to wait long for service. A brimming pot of tea would be set on the table, cups that had been warmed, and always some delightful sweet that we couldn't recognize, but that were as special as Mary.

Among our regulars were Dan and Alice Brusich and their two little fox terriers, who were always in need of care, nails trimmed if nothing else. The Brusich home, about eight miles north of Ketchikan, bordered a lovely cove adorned with clusters of islands. Dan had built a long dock extending out into the cove, where locals could rent space for their boats or seaplanes. Dan had a busy place, for it was the most sheltered spot along the Narrows. It was also the kind of spot Wally and I hoped someday we would find for ourselves. Dan and Alice often drove us out to their home when we had free time on a Sunday. It was good to have clients we could depend on seeing every trip. It gave us a sense of belonging.

There was still one person we hadn't met, one we very much wanted to meet. We'd caught glimpses of Betty King.

It would be difficult not to spot her. She had carrot-red hair and, even on the hottest day, wore a coat, a bright orange one that matched her hair. Betty King never walked alone. There were always five or six dogs on leashes dancing around her. She was extraordinary, to say the very least.

One day, as we were walking to the clinic, we saw her coming along the street toward us. I felt my heart quicken even as Wally squeezed my hand.

"We're in luck. We're going to meet her at last."

As we neared, she turned abruptly and crossed the street, a very deliberate maneuver. We were stunned.

"I feel like I've been stomped on," Wally said. "What is it about us she disapproves of? She hasn't even given us a chance to explain ourselves."

"I guess it's like Herb said. She takes her own sweet time to make up her mind."

"That I can understand, but to deliberately turn away from us! It's like she *has* made up her mind, and the way I see it, we don't set too well with her."

Wally said no more about it. I knew he was troubled and deeply hurt. He found it difficult to accept Betty King's rejection.

One afternoon, when Wally was out picking up a prescription at the drugstore, she came right into the clinic, leading a dog on a leash. Another dog was cradled in the arms of an elderly gentleman, who followed so closely in her footsteps I wondered how he avoided stepping on her heels. She hesitated just inside the door, seeming to question her action. The elderly gentleman with her was more confident.

"This son of—" He got no further.

Turning on him in shrill fury, Betty denounced him with a string of expletives that were as colorful as her dress. Then her voice softened. "Don't you dare talk like that in front of Mrs. Flynn. She's a lady."

Her arrival, her attitude, and her language had caught me off guard. I was confused, certainly relieved when Wally walked in the door.

For a moment he said nothing, as taken aback as I had been. He regained his composure and held out his hand.

"Mrs. King!" he said. "We've been hoping to meet you."

She inclined her head slightly, ignoring his hand, and I saw the flush mount his face. Her face was expressionless as she studied him. Then she spoke, weighing each word. "I have not liked you."

"I know. We've felt it. Would you care to tell us why?"

She nodded, then proceeded, her speech precise. Betty King was not one to bandy words. "Ketchikan is my town. I have many animals. People give me sick animals. I make them well. Then you come. You kill!"

I stifled a gasp, but Wally retained his composure. "I understand," he said. "We do put animals to sleep, but only if there's no alternative. If an animal is sick we try as hard as you do to make him well. But if an owner no longer wants an animal . . . well, you know what happens to animals here you weren't given a chance to adopt. They're taken out and shot."

She winced, then nodded. Taking courage from her silent admission, Wally continued. "Don't you think it is kinder to put them to sleep than to have them shot or let them suffer needlessly from sickness or injury when there is no hope of recovery?"

She nodded again. "So! I have come."

"And I thank you. I want us to be friends."

A faint smile relaxed the stern features of her face. "I think we are friends, but"—she hesitated—"doctors cost much money and . . . and I have so many."

"Forget the money. Just let us help."

Again the smile. "You are good people. I need your help. I will do what you say. Old Toby there" —she pointed to the dog in the old man's arms— "he won't eat. I have tried everything. He is very weak now. He needs more than I have to give him."

"He does," Wally agreed, taking him from the man, whom she had not bothered to identify, and laying him on the examination table. No one spoke while he made his examination, but Betty watched closely, her eyes anxious.

"It is not too bad," Wally said at last. "I will give him the medicine he needs, and you will give him the loving care. Together we will make him well."

For the first time Betty allowed a smile to have its way, and in spite of lines of age, she was beautiful. We had met her at last.

Chapter 12

The flight home, with a stop at Prince Rupert, brought a question from Harold. "Ever considered working here, Doc?"

"I've toyed with the idea," Wally admitted. "But I'm not licensed in British Columbia. I'd need a go-ahead from Immigration, too."

Harold shrugged. "Have a talk with Bert Glassey anyway. He's been taking care of animals here longer than he cares to remember."

Mr. Glassey had been a judge, whose love for animals compelled him to help them. A slight, grayed man in his seventies, he was eager, even anxious, to be relieved of those responsibilities. He'd kept at it, he told us, because veterinarians weren't interested in a town where there was no assurance they could make a living.

"There's a little of the materialistic in all of us," Wally conceded. "However, we do stop here. It wouldn't take much to persuade us to prolong our stay."

That was an understatement if I ever heard one. Wally would jump at a chance to work in Prince Rupert. It was all I could do to hold back the grin that was twitching at the corners of my mouth. (Wally, engaged in formal conversation with this pleasant, proper old English gentleman, was not the Wally I knew.) Mr. Glassey assured us that both the British Columbia Veterinary Association and Canadian Immigration would be cooperative. We left Prince Rupert with no promises given. In Wally's mind, it was settled.

In the meantime there was work waiting for us both in Seattle and in Friday Harbor. It was foxtail season in Friday Harbor. This obnoxious weed, its spears dried by the summer sun, is the bane of all animals. The spears puncture the flesh and travel, like a needle, following the path of least resistance. Not an animal came into our clinic that did not have one or many: in their ears, their noses, or just hanging on to their coats. If they were not shaken off, they worked their way along to a spot where they could enter.

"I've never seen it so bad," Wally observed. "Hate to suggest that people keep their pets penned up until the rains come and beat those damn spears into the ground, but it's about the only way. And that might not work. The wind blows them around. They can be picked up most anywhere."

He shook his head over our next case, an English setter. His master had taken him quail hunting in the cleared grassy areas of the island.

"Buzz is a mess," he told us.

It was not an exaggeration. Foxtails had worked between the toes of all four feet, some two and three foxtails crowding in against each other. All four feet were swollen and infected, discharging pus. We anesthetized him and went to work.

We could see some of the spears, and these were easily removed. The others had worked up the legs to a distance of five or six inches. Removing these required the use of an alligator, a delicate instrument with miniature jaws that, when manipulated correctly, would clamp over the spear. This is work that has to be done by feel alone. Wally would insert the alligator into the opening, gently probing until he felt the alligator butt up against the spear. When that spear was removed a search had to be made for others, for where one had entered others would follow.

Wally stood hunched over the table, flexing his shoulders occasionally to ease the strain. It was a hot day. Beads of perspiration formed on his forehead and trickled down his nose. With one hand I took a handerchief and wiped them away, careful to keep a steady hand on the leg he was working on.

"I think we've got them all," he said finally. "We'll get the two left feet bandaged. They were the worst. The other two should be okay."

By the time his master returned, Buzz had come out of the anesthetic, though he looked rather pathetic lying there on the floor with his two bandaged feet. His master leaned down and patted him on the head.

"Okay, Buzz boy? Guess we learned our lesson. No more hunting till those damn foxtails are gone from the fields. Thanks, Doc," he added. "We both appreciate you."

"Glad we got here to take care of it. A few days and he'll be as good as new," Wally assured him.

For Buzz it was not a matter of days—relief was immediate. His tail beat the floor in a happy rhythm. He allowed himself to be carried through the door; then he squirmed away and bounded down the street, running lightly on the two unbandaged feet.

Wally's grin was pure delight. "I'll be damned. Never before saw a dog run on just two legs on the same side. Remarkable!"

When Wally was not working he was studying. On our way back from Alaska he'd checked in Vancouver with Dr. Kenneth Chester, Registrar of the British Columbia Veterinary Medical Association. Dr. Chester had assured him that Prince Rupert was too small and too isolated to attract any of their members. They had no objection to his working there. That should have ended the matter, but it didn't. Wally wanted to become a member of their association, even though it was not required of him. I was not concerned with the upcoming exam, having gotten involved in something else, and quite against my will.

In late September I'd been approached to initiate a 4-H club dog obedience training program in Seattle. I knew nothing about training dogs, and protested. Wally insisted I could learn, and Maureen was positive there were kids at school who'd jump at the chance to enroll.

"I'll take a notice to school," she offered. "Lots of kids will come, I bet."

I groaned inwardly when Maureen took the notice to school, and I awaited the fateful day in a state of near panic. The school had cooperated, offering us the use of the school grounds for Saturday training sessions. The kids were there, holding every dog firmly on leash. I faced dogs and kids, my mouth dry, my throat constricted. My eyes swept the impatient lineup of dogs, ranging from a three-month-old dachshund to a dignified eight-year-old Irish setter, who sat apart from the others, disdainful of the yips of protest from animals unaccustomed to restraint. A Doberman and elkhound had taken an active dislike to each other, straining at their leashes. Either I controlled these animals or I'd have the wildest melee ever witnessed in one schoolyard.

"Separate those two," I called. "Take your positions at opposite ends of the line. If you don't make them know you're boss, they'll run you. Now! The first command is sit. Tighten up on your leashes. Push down on their haunches and give the command."

We were not immediately successful, but these kids were determined. I no longer felt panic. To the dogs, at first it had seemed a game, but, taking their cue from Spif (Maureen had worked hard to train her), they gradually responded. All, that is, except for George, a little dachshund, whose response to commands was to come later. Now he was running happily from one youngster to another, sniffing each one, seeming not to know, or care, who was his trainer. Eventually, however, he did learn, to a degree.

Of course, there were always one or two troublemakers, not necessarily always the same two, and at least one female in heat who had to be excluded temporarily. Then there were Saturdays when snow kept us off the school grounds. But for the most part it went well.

It had not gone so well for Wally. On his first attempt to pass the British Columbia exam, he failed. In January he tried again and made it. He was on top of the world, though I hardly noticed. My kids were keeping me busy.

National 4-H week had been set for March. It presented a

challenge they could not resist. Having decided on a demonstration in Lake City, our local shopping district, they worked hard to perfect their training program. As the time for the demonstration neared, a question arose.

"Who'd have us?" one of them asked.

"McKinnon's Furniture would be best," another speculated.

"Yeah! They've got that big showcase window. Naw! They'd never let us in . . . all that fancy furniture."

"Let's not give up before we even get started," I said. "We can at least ask."

"Yeah, but who?"

"Not me," one of the boys asserted. "I know what they'd say to me. 'You crazy, kid?' "

All eyes turned to me. I knew what they were thinking, and I knew they were right. It had to be me.

I approached the manager of McKinnon's with trepidation. I could see his resistance flare with my first words. I stood my ground.

"I know it sounds wild," I admitted, "but these are all Lake City youngsters. They've worked hard. I think they deserve the cooperation of Lake City merchants."

"That's all well and good, but why me?" he demanded. "I don't want to seem unfeeling, but dogs and furniture don't mix. Can't you have your show out on the sidewalk?"

"No, really. People jostling them! It would be impossible to control the dogs. If you could just move your furniture back a ways so we could have the front window. The dogs will be on leash."

"Good Lord, woman! Well, okay. If you've got nerve enough to ask, I guess I've got nerve enough to go along with it, but I don't mind telling you I have serious doubts about this whole affair."

The big day came. The manager didn't look exactly happy to see us, but the children were too excited to notice. The demonstration proceeded without incident until Susie came in with George. Somehow the leash slipped from her hand, and George, tail wagging his delight, darted in amid the expensively upholstered furnishings. With a wail of despair, Susie started after him.

My heart skipped a beat. "Dear Lord!" I'd have banned him from the show, only it would have broken Susie's heart. I looked at her now, white-faced, tears welling up in her eyes as she played hide-and-seek with George around a blue brocade davenport. If anything happened to that davenport! I caught a glimpse of the manager, his lips compressed into a hard, tight line. If he interfered before I did, it could only make matters worse.

"Susie! Stop! He thinks it's a game. Use your command."

Her voice quavered, but the command was firm. "Come!"

And he came, responding joyfully to his favorite command. I'd been holding my breath. With an almost audible sigh, I exhaled, glancing at the manager as I did so. He was exhaling, too. I had to give him credit. He simply shook his head.

There were no more problems until about four in the afternoon. Shad, the German shepherd, while waiting his turn, pulled to the side, sniffed the side of an upholstered rocker, and made a motion to lift his leg. The episode with George paled by comparison. He had merely wanted to play. Shad's natural inclination to relieve himself demanded prompt action.

"Shad! Sit!"

I hardly realized the command had come from me, but Shad sat. Another crisis had been averted.

Throughout the day the kids demonstrated the simple commands their dogs had learned. People came and went in front of our window, with approving faces. As the last kid and the last dog went out the door, the manager approached me.

"I didn't think I'd make it through this day," he confessed, "but I've actually enjoyed myself. Great bunch of kids! And I couldn't have asked for better advertising—all free, too."

Chapter 13

I was just hanging up the telephone receiver in the office when Wally walked into the room.

"Someone coming in?" he asked.

"Yes, Happy."

Wally chuckled. "Not so happy right now, I take it."

"Evidently not. Mr. Lewis said he'd disappeared, so he should be showing up here before long."

"Yeah. Listen for him, will you? I was going to ask you to give me a hand downstairs, but I'll get Tom."

Happy was a most unusual dog. The Lewis family was a large one, five children, and they all adored Happy. He adored them, too, although periodically their teasing and their rambunctiousness became too much for him. His skin would erupt in a mass of tiny red sores. The first time the family brought him in, we were uncertain as to the cause of these eruptions. We gave him medicated baths and, because he seemed more nervous than his condition warranted, some tranquilizing tablets. In a few days he was fine, and when the family came for him he greeted them exuberantly, his tail bopping the legs of the children, proof of his love.

We promptly forgot Happy, but Happy hadn't forgotten us. About a month later we heard soft whines and a scratching at the office door. When we opened the door, there was Happy. Alone! He bounded into the room, greeting us effusively.

"Where in thunder did you come from?" Wally asked him as he bent down to have a look at him. "Hmm! Broken out again, eh? Well, we'll give your family a call and see if they want us to treat you."

"So that's where he disappeared to," Mr. Lewis exclaimed when I got him on the phone. "I'm amazed he found you. And more amazed he didn't get himself killed dodging traffic all the way there. But as long as he's there, yeah, go ahead and treat him."

Happy had to have become expert at dodging cars, for he made the three-mile run frequently, and never once was hit. He was smart, too. He knew that after he'd seen us he always felt better. His problem was diagnosed as nervous dermatitis, brought on by the children he loved. His jaunts to the hospital became a matter of course, and the family ceased to worry when he disappeared. Mr. Lewis would get on the phone and simply say: "Happy's on his way. Take care of him."

And now Happy was on his way again. It wasn't long before I heard the familiar scratching at the door. I welcomed him as usual, petting him, calling him by name, and then I examined him more closely.

"Happy, you rascal, there's nothing wrong with you. What is this? Just a social call?"

Wally laughed when I told him. "Guess Happy thinks he has two families. Doesn't want to neglect us. I'll give the Lewises a call and tell them to come and get him."

Mr. Lewis was not upset. He chuckled. "Give him a treatment anyway. Maybe he feels it coming on. Wouldn't surprise me any. He may be just a mutt, but he's the smartest damn dog I ever owned."

As we worked over Happy, Wally became suddenly serious. "Work has sort of piled up on us, Chicken. I've been doing some thinking. There's enough work here to keep another man busy full time, and now that we're taking on Prince Rupert . . ." The words trailed off as he studied me, watching for my reaction.

I didn't answer at once. Ours had been a closed partnership. I wasn't sure I wanted to open it up to anybody else. Still, to be honest, I had to admit it had become a hassle to get another doctor to fill in for us when we were away. Johnny Bender wasn't always available, and, as Wally had said, there really was enough business for two men.

"Have anyone in mind?" I asked.

"Yes, Bob Harcus. He's worked with us enough to know our procedures and many of our clients. He's a good man."

"Okay, let's ask him."

The partnership with Dr. Harcus gave Wally time for other activities. He joined the Coast Guard Reserve and the Sheriff's Flying Squadron, taking part in search-and-rescue missions. We had long been members of the local Airplane Owners and Pilots Association. Elected to the presidency, Wally worked through them to have Friday Harbor designated a port of entry for seaplanes entering the U.S. from Canada. He saw the need for air-pollution control and campaigned for measures to achieve it.

"Honestly," I complained to him one day, "you're getting so involved we hardly have more than a nodding acquaintance anymore."

"Can't have that," he retorted with a grin, drawing me into the circle of his arms.

The ringing telephone interrupted. Wally picked up the receiver.

"Hey!" I heard him say. "This is great. Come on out to dinner."

"Dinner?" I questioned that before I even asked whom he'd invited. I'd always been cautious about whom we invited for dinner. A houseful of animals is risky insurance for gracious entertaining.

Wally laughed, and his eyes were beaming. "Don't worry. It's only Herb."

I still worried, but Herb was the same Herb. He enveloped Maureen in a bear hug, winning her completely. Spif demanded her share of attention, and Vicki sniffed at his pants leg and, satisfied, went back to her cushion. Minx rubbed against him, arching her back. Only Gardenia remained aloof, snappish eyes peering out from under a chair.

Age hadn't improved Gardenia's disposition or her behavior. She was quick and intelligent, especially adept at learning things I would rather she didn't learn. We loved her even when we wanted to throttle her. This evening I hoped her unexpected shyness would curb her more enterprising tendencies, but it was contrary to her nature to be still for long. A flurry of black-and-white, nails clicking across the floor, a quick flip with one curved nail, and the door to my pan cupboard swung open. She darted in, the pots and pans clattering as she squirmed among them.

"Gardenia," I muttered between clenched teeth, "come out of there."

She wouldn't, of course. I looked at Herb. His face was as red as mine, only he looked as if he were about to explode, and he did, in a howl of laughter.

"I'm sorry," he apologized. "Come on! I'll help you wash the dishes."

"You mean you're willing to stay to dinner?"

"Sure! Why not? I'm having a good time."

Shaking my head, I started hauling out the pans. Herb did help, talking at the same time with Wally, giving us all the latest news of Ketchikan.

I cooked the meal and served it without incident. Gardenia finally waddled out of the cupboard to beg for tidbits. It was a habit I frowned on. Spif, Vicki, Minx, all knew better than to beg, but a no to Gardenia was wasted breath. Her bad habit did serve a purpose this evening, however. It gave Herb an opportunity to make friends with her. Gardenia would never hold out against anyone who gave her what she wanted.

"I don't know whether she likes me or she's playing me for a sucker," Herb said with a grin, "but I'm willing to be accepted on any terms."

Later she climbed into his lap, wriggling sideways until the lap was arranged to her liking. An amused smile twitched at the corners of his mouth as he caressed the lovable black-and-white scamp.

"Quite a family, Doc. Quite a family!"

Chapter 14

If our family was demanding, our patients were equally so, and at the most inconvenient times. A month or so after Herb's visit, we began making plans for a flight to Prince Rupert. We went to bed early the night before we planned to leave, hoping for an early start the next morning. In the middle of the night I was awakened by persistent, calculated barks. I sat up in bed, rubbing my eyes, and awakening Wally as I attempted to climb over his hulking body.

"What's up?" His voice was groggy with sleep.

"It's lover boy."

"Oh! Well, I'll let him in."

"Never mind! I'm already up. Besides, it's my turn."

I went to the reception room and unlocked and opened the door. There was lover boy, a handsome liver-and-white setter, prancing on the walk, barks punctuating his demands.

"Spike! You get in here."

He sprang through the door, greeting me with moist, slobbery kisses. I pushed him aside.

"Spike! You shut up and settle down. All the kids are asleep." I glanced at my wristwatch. "Shame on you anyway. It's three in the morning. Come on now. Get into your kennel."

One kennel was expressly reserved for him, for he was an incurable romantic. After a night on the town, weary at last of philandering, he would invariably wind up at the hospital, demanding entry and a bed for the remainder of the night. His master didn't worry, having learned from experience where the wanderer could be found.

Though I sometimes complained that the animals, especially our own, were pushing us around, I wouldn't have had it otherwise. They did run the show!

When we arrived in Prince Rupert, Harold delivered us to the door of the shop that would serve as our clinic. He turned the key in the lock, and the door swung open. I gasped in disbelief. It was a tiny room with no windows. If it was privacy one wanted, certainly privacy could be had here. The shadows in that pitiful, unlit room seemed to reach out to us, belying the brightness of a hot July sun. In the middle of the room a single bulb was attached to an electric light cord dangling from the ceiling.

The men had to stoop to get in the door, and once inside, it was evident the ceiling was barely high enough to allow them to stand upright. When Wally turned on that one dim bulb, bundles of newspapers were revealed, stacked against the walls and scattered around the room.

"Sure not very damn elegant." Harold spoke for all of us.

Wally's lips were compressed into a tight line. "Well, at any rate, we can use the newspapers." Then he shook his head. "I don't know! With the two of us in here, a client, and an animal, it'll be damned cramped. Hope we won't have to use much ether. Liable to blow us the hell out of here."

Harold's easy grin had faded. "It's that bad? I'm sorry, Doc. When I put your ad in the paper, this room was offered, and I accepted it sight unseen."

It was bad. There were a few electric outlets, but there was no water at all. As I chewed at the tip of one finger, my mind flashed back to that cleaning shop in Petersburg where we had initiated our northern clinics. With a half smile and a wink, I reminded Wally, "No picnic!"

He managed a wry grin. "No picnic."

"Hell, Doc," Harold exploded, "don't quit on us. I'll get you water if I have to pack it myself."

"Who said anything about quitting?" Wally came back at him. "Let's get cracking. First off, let's get a bulb that will throw some light around here."

We did pack water, buckets and buckets. We got a basin for washup and a galvanized tub for the disposal of soiled water. Backbreaking work, but somehow we converted that dingy, pocket-sized room into a clinic. The inconveniences were many and annoying, but the clients came, indifferent to the surroundings.

"You never know what you can do until you have to face up to it," Wally commented at the end of the day. "I tell you, when I saw this damn room I felt like turning tail and getting the hell out of town. Back aches, though. Knew I wouldn't hit my head on the ceiling, but I couldn't rid myself of the feeling I would. Oh, well, come along. Let's have a look around town."

Unlike Ketchikan, whose business section covered several square blocks, Prince Rupert merchants had, for the most part, congregated along either side of one long street. A few Indians, their faces expressionless, leaned up against the buildings, but something was missing. Of course, the noise! All the taverns, or pubs, as they call them, were at the extreme end of the street. They stood wall to wall as if together they could defy the respectability of that one main street. We had passed several cafés on our tour and decided we were hungry.

"Hope you're in the mood for Chinese food," Wally remarked.

"I guess so. Come to think of it, I haven't seen anything but Chinese restaurants. How come, I wonder. So many Chinese people here, and none in Ketchikan."

"They worked on the railroad, I'd say. Prince Rupert is the end of the line. When the job was finished, they stayed."

"And opened Chinese restaurants," I finished for him. "Okay. I'm for Chinese food. How about you?"

Word of our clinic spread, and patients came from as far as Terrace, a hundred miles away over a dusty, rutted road.

"Something, isn't it?" Wally observed. "Wonder if I'd drive over that road if I was in their shoes. Oh, I suppose I would. The way people look at you, though, makes you want to be as good as they think you are."

"You are!" I thought as I clipped away at the matted coat of a cocker.

Wally left me to check on phone calls. We had a house call, he said when he returned, at a place down near Seal Cove. Although we discouraged house calls, there would always be exceptions. The woman who called Wally had said her husband would pick us up.

Very soon a perky individual appeared in an old pickup truck to chauffeur us to what turned out to be an old army barracks. He pulled into the yard with a flourish. Geese shrilled in protest; dogs, cats, even rabbits scattered in all directions.

"Take it easy," Wally protested.

"Aw! Don't worry. Ain't never hit one yet."

A woman appeared in the doorway of the barracks. "Shame on you, Lee," she reproached our driver. "You got no call to scare folks thataways. He always does it," she apologized. "Don't know what gets into him. Well, come on into the kitchen, folks. I'm Lucy. I'll pour you some coffee, and maybe you can help me figure what to do about my family here."

A rather plain woman, I decided as we followed her in, face, figure, and dress all seeming to blend. Nice and pleasant, but a very average person, one you would meet and then forget.

As she ushered us into the kitchen she swatted tolerantly at a cat perched on the kitchen table. "Git you, Henrietta! I've told you before, stay off the table. Made a mistake on this one," she said turning to us. "Named her Henry. Ha! She showed me."

She pulled a chair from the table, dislodging another cat. "Git down, Lizzie. Pretty, isn't she? But, dear, dear, the size of her litters. I really don't know how many cats I have around here."

That I could believe. One was slinking across the top of a

cupboard. A black cat peered around from behind the door.

"Doctor," she went on, "do you think if I had some of them taken care of . . . that operation, whatever you call it, that maybe there wouldn't be so many?"

"It would help some, all right," Wally agreed. And I saw that he was not amused by the scene but was as serious as she was.

"Not that I don't love them all, you understand, but it's hard to keep on familiar terms with so many."

I was inclined to disagree. One pretty ginger kitten leaped into my lap, mewing affectionately, pushing up under my arm, causing me to almost spill my coffee. It would be difficult not to be on familiar terms with these cats.

"The trouble is," she continued, her mouth drawn into a pucker, "I don't know which ones to have this done to, poor dears. Some are a whole lot pregnant and some maybe just a little bit. I'm not sure, you know, the ones that are just a little bit, that is. If they're going to be mothers, I couldn't interfere."

It was evident she was disturbed about the morality of calling us in, but Wally was understanding, answering her questions, explaining away her doubts and fears. Henrietta, of course, could not be taken. She was expecting almost any day, and Lizzie also was quite pregnant, but Clara, the one in my lap, had no such excuse. Lee came in with some wooden crates. With a few slats nailed across the top, Clara was secure, although visibly annoyed. I could see Lucy's distress as she clasped and unclasped her hands, but from somewhere deep inside her she summoned up the courage to go ahead with her plan.

"There's more," she said. "If we just walk down the hall, they'll come. We were so fortunate, Lee and I, to be able to get this old barracks. So many rooms!"

And so many closed doors! I began to wonder, as she opened one after another, what we would find behind the next. One room housed two mother rabbits and their large families. In another, a collie barked a warning, nuzzling her puppies. I counted seven sable-and-white babies. Shrill peeps greeted us with the opening of yet another door, and a mother hen clucked to her brood of downy yellow chicks. How could she keep this incompatible collection all living peaceably under one roof?

We had, by this time, selected five females for surgery and, with some persuasion, three males. Lee, running back and forth along that long hall, dragging his boxes, made certain they did not escape to hiding places known only to themselves.

Lucy paused at another door. Quickly she scanned the hall. "Good! No cats!"

As she opened the door we were greeted by a burst of music. There were chirps and trills and songs of pure joy, and, all about us, the flutter of wings. Canaries and parakeets in all shades of blue, green, and yellow. They came to light on her shoulder, or on the top of her head. She would catch one in her hands, kiss the feathered head, and set it free. Tiny frame houses with slanting roofs lined the room. Most of the oc-cupants flew free, lighting in branches that were nailed to stands.

We followed Lucy around the room as she stopped to caress one, then another of her birds, calling many by name. She stopped at one small house.

"Are you home, darling?" she called, peering in through the circular doorway. "Ah, there you are! Come say hello to the doctor. She's going to have babies," Lucy announced happily.

"Do you raise them to sell?" It was an obvious question, yet the expression on her face changed from gentleness to de-fiance.

"Maybe I might sell one, if I'm real sure it will have a happy home, but I'm not anxious to sell. They need love to be happy."

"How many birds do you have in this room?" I persisted.

"Over a hundred, I guess." It was a reluctant admission, as if she felt I were criticizing her.

She opened the door and then closed it quickly after us,

more to keep the cats out than to keep the birds in, I suspected, for not one bird had attempted to escape. My admiration for this woman was profound.

"How do you ever manage to care for so many?" I asked.

There had been no unpleasant odors in any of the rooms. There were recent droppings, but no dried excrement left lying to soil the floor. The water bowls were filled with fresh water.

"I don't do anything else," she admitted. "I don't care to do anything else. Lee helps me when he isn't working, but mostly I do it myself."

There was still defiance in her voice, but I understood her now, understood her aversion to surgery, her reluctance to take from even one of her creatures any part of the fullness of life. Here was a truly happy woman. She was ideally suited for the work to which she had dedicated herself.

How, I wondered, could I ever have thought this woman was plain, or average? The warmth in her voice when she spoke to one of her creatures, the depth of the love that shone from her eyes, the gentleness of her hands as she fondled her beautiful birds, all bespoke a woman who was anything but average. She glowed, and I basked in that glow.

She let us leave with her cats, secure in their boxes, but there was a sadness in her eyes that told us she was not wholly persuaded she had made the right decision.

"Remarkable woman!" We were back at our clinic, but Wally seemed not to see me, his face a brown study. "We won't find many like her."

Like Betty King, too, I thought. Alike yet so unalike. Betty, loud, harsh, flamboyant in language and dress. Lucy, quiet, demure, almost nondescript, but so lovely. I loved them both, though I knew so little about either. We had learned early not to question clients about their background. Our business was to treat animals, not to probe into the private lives of our clients. Some undoubtedly had reasons for wanting their pasts forgotten. At any rate, since we held to a strictly cash basis, there was no reason for clients to furnish us with either references or background.

Lucy, however, remained in my thoughts long after we had returned her cats.

Before we left Prince Rupert we had another house call. It was within a few blocks of our clinic, so we walked, carrying our bag. The woman had given few details over the phone. She had a fox terrier, old and sick, she wanted put to sleep.

She met us at the door dressed in pink cotton pajamas. A white scarf was wrapped around her head like a turban. Her face was streaked with tears, which she dabbed at with a wad of handkerchief clutched in one hand.

"Oh, Do-o-octer!" she wailed as she led us into the living room, where a small white dog lay on a scarlet cushion. He offered no resistance to Wally's gentle examination.

"There's no point in letting him suffer more," Wally told the weeping woman. "At his age we could prolong his life for only a few days at best. I think you were resigned to his going to sleep when you called me. Would you like to wait in another room?"

"Oh, no, Doctor, I'm not leaving him until it's over. But don't do it yet. I want my husband here."

He came in reluctantly. He was a big, heavy man, and his face was flushed. He shifted uncomfortably from one foot to the other. This scene was obviously one he would have preferred to avoid.

As we prepared the injection, the woman's anguished wails increased in volume. I bit my lip, but Wally's eyes said "Steady," and I nodded. Then the wails stopped, the sudden silence almost more disturbing than the wailing. I glanced up, wondering what it could mean. She had turned to her husband, who stood rigid, his eyes focused straight ahead.

"Damn you!" she shrilled. "You're in the presence of death. Show a little respect. Bow your head."

He obeyed, his face a deep crimson. Again my eyes sought Wally's. His lips moved soundlessly. "Ready?"

I nodded, my hand tight on the vein. As the needle went in, a screech filled the room. I dropped the leg, but it didn't matter. The poor tired body had gone to its last sleep without even a quiver.

"Is he dead?" the woman demanded.

"Yes, he's gone," Wally assured her. "No more suffering."

"My God!" she marveled. "He never made a sound. How could you do it so easy?" She turned to her husband. "Pete, go get the casket." He left without a word, looking relieved to be excused. "We have the grave ready," she said.

She was all business now, not in the least distraught, which was more than I could say for myself. I was glad to go out that door, out into the dark silent night, glad to feel the cool sea breeze on my cheek. My hand sought Wally's.

We'd come to the end of our long list of appointments. Our bags had been stowed away in the pigeon, and we stood on the ramp exchanging a last few words with Harold.

"Next time, Doc, you'll have the biggest damn room in town, running water and all the conveniences."

"I'll hold you to it." But Wally was laughing, and I suspected he hadn't found that little room too objectionable after all. It had presented a challenge, and that he couldn't resist.

I was on the pontoon, preparing to climb into the pigeon, when another plane taxied up to the ramp. The door was flung open and the pilot jumped out.

"Glad I caught you, Doc. Just came up from Buttedale. They want you to stop on your way down. Have three or four cats that are overpopulating their establishment. I told them you could fix that."

"Can do!" Wally agreed with a jaunty salute. Harold pushed us out from the ramp and we were on our way. I turned in my seat.

"Happy?"

"You better believe it! You know," he mused, "the work load seems to increase with each trip. Working out like this is the greatest thing that could have happened to us. In the city, people can always find another veterinarian. Up north here, it's just us, and people are so damn glad to see us."

Chapter 15

I felt good as I walked along the hotel corridor in Toronto. The convention was over and we would be going home. We were so far east, Wally suggested, why not fly on to New York City? I didn't answer at once, recalling my reaction when he'd first suggested we fly to Toronto to attend the National Veterinary Convention.

"In a seaplane?"

"Why not? You'll be the first woman to cross the continent on pontoons. Doesn't that excite you?"

"It does not. There's too much dry land in between to suit me."

Though he'd gotten out maps and pointed out seaplane facilities across the country, I wanted no part of it. Then something happened back there in Seattle that changed my mind. Vicki, thirteen years old now, had developed bladder stones. She survived the surgery, but the tired old body had no spark. In a few days she was gone. I had been the one then to push for the Toronto flight . . . anything to bring the light back into Wally's eyes. The plans did excite him, and then, after the grief of losing Vicki became less poignant, he decided we had to have another Vicki.

The new Vicki took over with the same arrogance as her predecessor, and for the first time in her tempestuous life, Gardenia practiced tolerance. She had missed the old Vicki, sniffing around the apartment in search of her, glaring at us with condemning eyes, as though we were in some way responsible for the empty bed. Now here was a new Vicki, teasing, annoying, yet Gardenia adored her. She scolded her, mothered her, nudged her to bed at the proper time, covering her with that broad black-and-white tail. Vicki resisted at first, but soon came to accept the discipline of her foster mother. They were inseparable.

And so we had made the trip east. My mind skimmed over those four days: the flight through the Cascade Mountains and on across eastern Washington State, the hot July winds funneling small whirlwinds from the plowed fields below us. We'd stopped at Coeur d'Alene, Idaho, and a thunderstorm had pummeled us at Flathead Lake, where we'd spent our first night. I recalled the trouble we had taking off from the Missouri River at Fort Peck, Montana, with sandbars and a bridge barring our way. I saw again the lonely prairies of Montana, a state that it seemed to take forever to cross.

But then I smiled, remembering the green farmlands east of the Fort Peck Reservoir in Montana. We had been flying at an altitude of three thousand feet to avoid some of the turbulence caused by winds stirring the hot dry earth. Over the farmlands we dropped to one thousand feet, watching the farmers till their soil, watching the cattle in the fields lazily switching their tails to ward off flies. I had wished our pigeon had been a helicopter so that we might linger awhile.

We'd spent that second night at Devils Lake, North Dakota. At noon on the third day out we stopped for lunch at Lake Bemidji in Minnesota. From there on the country was green and wooded and there were many lakes. It was pleasant flying. That night we stayed on lakeshores at Boulder Junction, Wisconsin.

Fog had plagued us the morning of the fourth day as we flew along the narrow strip of land between Lake Michigan and Lake Superior. We were heading for Sault Sainte Marie, where we were to report to Canadian Customs. Sault Sainte Marie is actually two cities, one American, one Canadian, located on either side of the river. Our radioed instructions from the American tower were to land by the ferry dock on the Canadian side. The dock was easy to spot, for the ferry was in, but there was no ramp for seaplanes.

"We'll pull up on the riverbank," Wally decided. "Hop down on the pontoon, Chicken, and watch for any hidden obstacles."

I hopped down, but I didn't watch. People on the dock were waving and shouting. I waved and shouted, too, until I suddenly realized they were not waving. They were pointing.

"Stop!" I yelled to Wally.

Too late! Already the pigeon had come to rest, teetering on a rock just below the water's surface. Wally leaned out the door.

"Well?"

"It's a rock wall. I think I can touch bottom. Maybe I can wiggle us loose. Guess everyone's expecting a show anyway," I concluded wryly, glancing at the people who had left their cars to crowd along the railing.

Rolling up my jeans, I lowered myself into the water, keeping a firm grip on the pontoon in case I had misjudged the depth. The water was up to my jeans and my legs were still dangling. I hesitated, then slid in up to my waist, and my toes dug into the sandy bottom. I edged along the pontoon, wiggling the pigeon back and forth on her rocky perch. As she slid free, a cheer went up from the watching crowd.

"The seaplane ramp's downriver," someone shouted.

"Can you head us out?" Wally called to me.

I inched in between the two pontoons and pushed. Slowly the pigeon swung around. I held her steady while Wally flipped the propeller, then pulled myself up, planted both feet firmly on the pontoon, and grasped the wing strut with both hands. Wally glanced my way, and I nodded. Giving it full throttle, he pulled us out around the ferry. I took in stride the spray that shot over me. Past the ferry, he eased off and I scrambled into the cabin.

"A mite wet, I'd say," he observed, a twinkle in his eyes.

Flying at fifty feet off the water, we soon spotted a dock. "Ha!" Wally exclaimed. "There's even a seaplane here."

He edged in, and I jumped for the dock, rope in hand. As Wally got out of the pigeon, his eyes rested on me.

"Better put your shoes on."

"What possible difference can shoes make?"

An officer was striding down the dock. I ran to meet him, barefoot, wet, and mussed, but happy. Canada at last!

"Are you in trouble?" he asked, puzzled.

"No," Wally replied. "We're just checking in for Customs inspection."

"You can't check in here. This is a Government dock." His eyes flicked over me, and the official expression relaxed. "Wait here. I'll give Customs a call."

Customs responded. We found the seaplane ramp still four miles on downriver. After obtaining gas, we hopscotched in the fog over the islands of Georgian Bay, then headed inland, arriving at Lake Ontario's shores just after sunset. A million lights gleaming wanly in the dusk assured us we were approaching Toronto.

And now Wally wanted to fly on to New York City. Did I want to? Not really—but I knew that I would.

We could see all the way across Lake Ontario when we set out the next morning. Our first stop would be Youngstown, New York, on the St. Lawrence River, where we were to clear with American Customs. The town was only a dot on our map, and from the air appeared not much larger. Wally frowned as he studied our landing area.

"The way the wind's picked up it's going to be tricky, especially with all those boats cluttering up the river."

"Maybe seaplanes don't ordinarily land here," I suggested.

"Maybe not. But they're expecting us, so we'd better get down."

The dock proved to be a wharf, a wretched affair for a seaplane, so high our wing barely cleared. A couple of men caught our wing tip, struggling against the wind to hold us in. Whatever made me think I could help? I braced my foot against a piling, and one of the men, kneeling to reach my outstretched hand, pulled me up onto the wharf. Wally turned from the Customs official.

"Get back down there," he said. "We're taking right off."

Contrarily, I waited for the roar of the engine before catching the wing strut to swing down. The men gave the wing a flip heading us out from the wharf. The flip flung me hard against the strut. There was a stab of pain in my rib area, but I clung to the strut until my feet touched the pontoon. Then I reached for the door, pushing against the wind to open it. Wally's voice was impatient.

"Quit stalling. Let's get the hell out of here."

As I pulled myself into the cabin, the pain came again. Then I sneezed. It brought an involuntary cry, and I clutched at my side.

"What's that all about?" Wally demanded.

"Guess I got a chill from this open window." I closed the window and wrapped myself in a sweater.

That night in our hotel room at Seneca Lake I edged into bed, thankful Wally was out of the room. If he knew I was hurt, he'd likely send me packing. We had started this trip across the continent together, and I intended we'd finish together.

But the next day in New York City, as we walked and walked, all I could think of was home. New York City did not thrill me. It was too hot. There were too many people, all of them in such a great hurry.

That night in our hotel room, Wally heard me gasp when I tried to lie down.

"Still feeling the effects of that sneeze? Could be pleurisy. Maybe you should see a doctor."

"No! Honest, I'm okay."

His "Hmm!" was noncommittal, but the next day he put an end to our sightseeing.

Our flight from New York City took us north along the Hudson River. The haze that had enveloped the city gave way to the sun, highlighting a panorama of wooded hills and shimmering lakes. We were going home. Home! Round Lake, Rochester, Toronto, Parry Sound, and Georgian Bay, again plagued by fog.

Wally worried. "All this island-hopping over the bay is playing hell with our gas supply. If we make it to Sault Sainte Marie we'll be damn lucky."

He took the pigeon up another thousand feet to give us the advantage of a long glide. I watched uneasily, straining for a first glimpse of the ramp. Even as I spotted it, our engine sputtered and died, but our glide carried us right to the ramp. The attendant shook his head as he caught our wing tip. "You want gas, I take it!" he said.

At Sault Sainte Marie there was Customs and Immigration again, twice, out of Canada, into the States. On the American side there was no ramp, and the rocky river bottom thwarted our efforts to pull to shore. About twenty feet out, a boulder protruded from the water.

"We'll nudge up to it," Wally decided. "Get a rope on the strut, Muscles. You can sit on the boulder and hold the pigeon in while I wade to shore."

"Honestly!" I grumbled. "If this isn't the darndest place for getting in and out of a country."

There I sat while Wally waded to shore and while the Customs officer waded back with him to have a peek into the plane.

Still so far from home! It seemed we'd never get across that vast expanse of land, but when we reached Fort Peck Reservoir, Washington State seemed not too distant. The day was too hot, though, the air was muggy, and the words of the attendant at the reservoir disturbing.

"Sure as shooting there'll be thunderstorms this afternoon." The sun beguiled us the full ninety-mile length of the reservoir, and I began to think the attendant had been wrong. But as we entered the narrow Missouri River canyon, clouds heavy with a burden of rain piled up on either side of us. Thunder boomed, lightning struck all around us, and the rain spilled down. The pigeon bucked and twisted in the clutches of the wind. It was no more than I had experienced many times on our flights to Alaska. This time, however, there was a difference. I had, rather successfully, I felt, been concealing the pain in my side. Concealment was no longer possible. I gasped and sobbed, clutching my side. Wally looked at me in alarm.

"I didn't realize the pain was so bad. Try to hang on, Chicken. I can see the rim of the sun up ahead."

How I welcomed the sight of that muddy riverbank at Fort Benton! Wally circled the little airfield, and a car sped down to the river to meet us. I couldn't get to the hotel fast enough. All I wanted was to crawl into bed. Wally's arm supported me as we walked into the lobby of the hotel. The clerk was apologetic but firm. There was a farmers' convention in progress, and not a spare room in town.

Wally persisted. There had to be one room. There was, the clerk admitted, but it had no windows. At Wally's insistence, he escorted us up a flight of stairs and unlocked a door. It was like walking into a well-stoked furnace.

"We'll take it," Wally said. "Leave the door open so some air can get in. We'll go out for supper."

We had our meal. We lingered over coffee, stalling for time. The café was closing, and we were out in the street. The stars shone bright and the night air was cool. In our room the night air had made no difference.

"We'll leave the door open," Wally said. "Maybe it won't be too bad."

His rhythmic snores soon filled the room and rumbled down the hall. I couldn't breathe; then my nose started to bleed. I got up to wash the blood away, and my eyes fell on the blankets we'd tossed aside. I made up a bed on the floor in front of that open door, with my pillow right out in the hall.

We needed no call to awaken us. No one could oversleep in that room, even with his head in the hall. And a night on the floor hadn't helped my side. Wally suggested again that I see a doctor, but all I wanted to do was get home.

Seattle! Lake Washington! How lovely the homes surrounding it were. Nothing we'd seen could compare. I called Maureen from the air harbor.

"Mom!" she cried. "Hurry and come home."

Minutes later, at the animal hospital, she ran to greet us, throwing her arms around us. Grandma came to the door.

"Coffee's ready. And the animals know you're here. They've gone crazy."

Maureen grabbed a bag, then turned to see me lagging behind. "What's the matter, Mom? You walk kind of funny."

"She does," Wally agreed. "Darn woman won't tell me a thing. You and Bob take her to the doctor while I get unpacked."

When we returned, no explanation was needed. "You're taped!" Wally exclaimed. "Broken ribs. Sure, I wanted you to make the trip, but not that way. Now will you tell me what happened?"

Chapter 16

It was Christmas Eve. Gift wrap and colorful ribbons were scattered everywhere. Were there only three of us? We seemed to be forever walking in on each other. Mysterious packages would be snatched up and held behind one's back. There was a kind of happy desperation in our attempts to avoid each other. In the midst of all this confusion the bell rang in the reception room. Maureen ran to see and was back in a few minutes with an odd expression on her face.

"It's a little boy. His garter snake is sick."

"Garter snake!" I snorted. "On Christmas Eve?"

"Well, now," Wally rationalized, "I guess a garter snake has as much right to be sick as anyone. Want to help, Maureen?"

I was glad to have the two of them out of the way. Now I could wrap those special gifts. I'd barely finished when they were back.

"What was the matter with the thing?"

"Oh, Mom! Poor little snake. It's not a thing."

"Of course it isn't," Wally concurred. "Too many Christmas goodies forced on him, I suspect. We got a little medicine down him with an eyedropper. He should perk up."

"I hope so. He was kinda cute."

"Maureen!"

"I know, Mom. No more pets! Anyway, a snake probably wouldn't get along with Gardenia or Minx."

"Or with me, either," I assured her.

"Okay, Mother dear!" Wally was laughing. "No snakes."

His sympathies, I knew, were with Maureen. There was no creature that didn't delight or intrigue them. In our practice there was no monotony. We'd had a sea gull with a broken wing, a duck who'd been bitten by a dog, a monkey that threw to the floor everything that wasn't nailed down or hastily removed and secured behind locked doors. Then there was the honey bear, a lovable little kinkajou that delighted in swinging from one of us to the other, wrapping its long tail around our arms. The ocelot, on the other hand, was a cantankerous creature, frustrating even to her owner, who handled her with leather gloves. My introduction to her was startling. She escaped her owner in the reception room and sprang onto my back, the sharp nails digging into my flesh as she climbed up and over my shoulder.

Although we loved all these creatures, it was the little red Pekingese, Boo, who most aroused our admiration. This feisty fellow was a scrapper. Size made no difference to him. He'd tackle anything from a fox terrier to a German shepherd with a determination to win that was unshakable. He'd been in the hospital any number of times with wounds varying from minor to critical, but none so critical as those he sustained the week after Christmas.

"What do you think, Doc?" Mr. Noble laid the still body on the examination table. "I'm afraid he's done for this time. I can feel his heart beating, but he hasn't stirred since I found him lying out on the boulevard. I've tried to keep him fenced in, but he manages to dig out. I don't know what he tackled this time."

"By the looks, it was a shepherd or a boxer, the very least," Wally said, bending over to examine him more closely. "I'd say whichever it was took him by the head and shook the hell out of him. Look here. He's got a hole on either side of his head. You can almost look through from one side to the other.

And that one eye's had it. It will have to come out . . . if he lives."

"If he lives! Yeah! I get it. Do what you can, Doc. I've gotten so mad at him myself at times I could have almost killed him. But he's got the guts of a . . . Doc! Dammit. I love him."

For the better part of a week we weren't sure Boo would make it. He came around enough to follow our movements with his good eye. The holes in his head had to be cleaned and irrigated and packed with healing ointments any number of times a day. He took it stoically, wihout benefit of anesthesia, which we hesitated to use, considering his weakened condition. He seemed indifferent to pain. He should have died that first week, but he would not. His will to live was as strong as his will to fight.

"A dog with that much spunk deserves to live," Wally declared. "We're going to pull him through, Chicken."

A couple of more weeks and he was up and running around, eating well, and the flesh was filling in those holes on either side of his head. I anticipated Wally's next move and I dreaded it, while knowing it had to be. I'd always been squeamish about eyes. To me, the worst that could happen would be to lose an eye. I could have avoided that surgery— Bob would have helped—but my admiration for Boo was so profound that I was determined to see him through this last step in his recovery.

The surgery wasn't as repulsive as I'd expected. There was little loss of blood. Almost before I realized it had happened, Wally had the eye out. He handed it to me. My stomach was still queasy, but I took it and forced myself to look. It was round and hard, like a marble, bearing little resemblance to the pliant, yielding orbs that looked back at me in the mirror.

I had dreaded, too, seeing that empty space where an eye should have been, but when Wally removed the sutures and the hair grew back over that fine line where the incision had been made, I hardly noticed one eye was missing. Certainly

Boo didn't seem to notice. He was as happy and as full of spice and ginger as he'd ever been. When Mr. Noble came to pick him up, he bounced all over the place, snorting his delight through his funny flat nose.

"This calls for a celebration," Wally declared. "I'll take you to a show. Want to go, Maureen?"

"Uh-uh! I'm loaded with schoolwork. You guys go ahead."

I went, although reluctantly.

I knew what to expect. Wally's keen sense of observation noted things that escaped a less critical mind, observations he didn't keep to himself. As the hero and heroine embraced, there was a nudge in my side and Wally's hoarse whisper came through the darkness.

"Odd I never ever noticed that melanoma behind his left ear."

"Shh!" came from either side, and the couple in front of us turned and glared. For a few minutes the screen lovers were permitted to romanticize without extraneous comment, but Wally couldn't refrain for long.

"Just as I thought," he hissed. "She's got false teeth."

We managed to see the show through without being evicted from the theater, but I was relieved, as I'm sure those around us were also, when we got up to leave.

Maureen was ready for bed when we got home. "How was the show?" she asked, stifling a yawn.

"Terrific! A hot romance between a hero with a melanoma behind his ear and a heroine with false teeth."

She giggled. "Sounds great. Well, it wasn't exactly dull around here, either. Come see what I took in."

She led the way to the kennel room and, opening the door of one of the kennels, took out a cardboard box. A robin, a little wobbly on its feet, huddled in one corner.

"The woman said it flew into her front window. Said she heard a plop, but didn't think anything about it. She thought it was dead when she went out later and happened to see it. It was only stunned, though, and I don't think anything's broken. I got a hot water bottle and put that blanket over it.

You're coming along okay, aren't you, little robin?" she finished.

"I'd say so," Wally agreed. Then he chuckled, but his voice told us he meant it when he added, "If there's one thing a doctor needs when he goes out to celebrate, it's a daughter who tends his business for him."

Chapter 17

Sullivan Bay was the start and finish of each northern flight. It was there our work began; it was there we would finish it up. That Sullivan Bay had a population of only three, compared to the eight thousand of Ketchikan or Prince Rupert, did not matter. Skippy and the cats, whose numbers fluctuated according to the number of kittens that could be given away, ranked right along with all the other animals we treated in the course of our travels. We checked them routinely each time we stopped. We loved all animals but, as is natural, we had favorites. Skippy was one of them, maybe because we saw him more often, maybe because when we sat with the Collinsons, enjoying coffee, Skippy was always at our feet, adoring us.

Skippy was growing old. When we stopped in on our way home after our September clinics, the grin with which Rod always greeted us as he hauled in the pigeon was replaced by a worried frown.

"Troubles, Rod?" Wally asked.

"Yeah. Skippy has a lump on his back."

"Let's have a look."

Skippy had several smaller lumps besides. "But it's nothing to be worried about," Wally assured Rod. "They're fatty tumors. Sometimes come with old age. I think we should remove that big one, though! Is there someplace where we can set up for surgery?"

"There's the cabin I'm building for myself. It's not finished. Couple of sides to put up yet, but the roof's on."

"It'll do." Wally glanced at the sky. Black clouds were boiling up to the north. "Let's get right at it. Looks like we're in for a squall before long."

We set up our surgery near an open side, to take advantage of the light. Before we had finished, the black clouds descended on Sullivan Bay with a full load of rain. Wally bent over Skippy, straining to see.

"Would a flashlight help, Doc?" Rod asked.

"Yes. Get one."

The squall was a rough one. Rain beat in at us, and our cabin, on its foundation of logs, swayed and jerked as angry waves pounded our floating village. But with Rod holding the flashlight, we removed the tumor and sutured the incision. Then, throwing a blanket over Skippy, we made a dash for the kitchen, where Myrt was preparing supper.

"I'm glad that operation's over with," she said. "I ran by after it began to rain. If you could have seen yourselves! The cabin was so black inside. All I could see was the gleam of the flashlight and three figures bent over a lump in the middle of the table. It was positively eerie."

At the sound of her voice Skippy raised his head, then let it drop, as if the effort to hold it up were too great. He wasn't long in coming out of the anesthesia. His eyes still wore that groggy look when he wobbled over and lay down at Wally's feet.

Wally grinned as he leaned over to pet him. "Not the fanciest setup in the world, old boy, but you got as good a treatment as any. You'll do okay."

Skippy was out on the float to greet us on our trip up the following June. Rod was there, too, of course.

"You know, Doc, he doesn't even have a scar where you made the incision. Man! That was beautiful. We've got another problem now, though."

"Let's have it."

"Well, do you remember us telling you about that old

hermit that lives around the bend? He sneaks in here once in a while for groceries when he's sure no strangers are around. I go down to check on him as often as I dare, though he doesn't much like being bothered."

"I do recall some talk about him. Odd we haven't spotted his house as we've come in."

"You wouldn't unless you were looking for it, Doc, and then you might miss it. It's just a shack, and pretty well hidden in the trees, but he's got a dog, a kind of special dog. The old man rows around a lot. He found this dog about ten years ago sitting on a reef out in the channel. We all figured the dog must have fallen from some passing troller and swum to that reef."

Wally nodded.

"Well, anyway, last time I was down there Blackie's ears stunk so bad I could hardly hang around. I took a look in them, though, and they're a mess . . . all pussy. Old Mr. Nesbit doesn't talk much, but he knows you come around. He told me he wished you'd fix Blackie, only he said he didn't have any money. He really loves that dog. I told him you'd take care of him, Doc."

"You get us there, Rod. We'll take care of it."

Rod took us in his speedboat to the old man's house—a hermit's house in every sense of the word, grayed and weather-beaten, with sagging steps and cracked windows. The old man met us at the door. He was as grayed and weather-beaten as the house, with thinning gray hair, and faded blue eyes peering out from a grayed and wrinkled face. He gave me a feeling of unreality, as if it were an apparition standing there in the door.

The grayness extended to the interior as the sun struggled to penetrate the collection of cobwebs that covered the windows. It was a house without paper or paint. There was not a chair that didn't hold something—a frayed Indian sweater, tattered books and magazines. A bathtub that had never known running water was thick with dust, a catchall for pots and pans. The table was covered with newspapers, some dated ten years previous. There was one single exception to the gray monotone, a single white circle where his plate lay on the table.

Rod's announcement that we had come to help Blackie brought only a nod. Shoving magazines from a chair, he lifted the unresisting dog up onto it. The dog's body trembled, anticipating the unknown, but his sense of obedience kept him glued to the chair. His muzzle had grayed with the years, but the shiny black coat bespoke his master's love and care. The diet of the dog had obviously taken precedence over the diet of the master.

The ears were ulcerated and painful. Blackie winced, but he didn't cry out. The old man maintained his stoic silence, even when Wally handed him several medications and instructed him in their use. Though he followed us to the door, watching as we climbed back into the boat, not even a wave of the hand acknowledged we'd been there.

"He really appreciated it, Doc." Rod's voice was apologetic.

"I know. Check on him, Rod. Make certain he follows those instructions."

We didn't see the old hermit or the dog when we came back down from our northern clinics, but Rod assured us the ears were much improved. In September, however, as we taxied up to the float, the old hermit came rowing alongside us. Blackie was with him. No word was spoken, but a smile brightened the wrinkled face and a hand was raised in salute. In his way he had said thank you.

Chapter 18

I knew something was wrong the minute Wally walked into the kitchen. It wasn't just the telegram he held in his hand, but the look on his face. He was stunned!

"What is it?" I asked.

"Harold. He's gone."

"Gone?" I repeated.

He was incapable of answering. I took the telegram and read for myself. Viv's message read that Harold was dead. While flying in snow-covered areas, delivering supplies to isolated mines, he had run into a whiteout, that perfect blending of clouds and snow that obliterates the horizon, and his plane had crashed.

Losing Harold had a profoundly sobering effect. We'd raced through life with little or no thought for the future, as if we'd go on forever flying those channels to Prince Rupert and Ketchikan, relegating to an uncertain future our dreams for a home somewhere in that vast wilderness we roamed so freely. Now the search became paramount.

Our initial hopes centered on Clowholm. The homeward trek from Alaska had never failed to include a few days with Al and Lavone Taylor. We were the first there in the spring, the last to leave in the fall. We discussed with Al the possibility of purchasing a bit of his land. Unfortunatly, civilization was catching up with Clowholm. British Columbia Electric planned to build a dam to generate more power for distant communities. Before too many summers, the rising waters of the lake would engulf the lodge and those two small cabins.

Our thoughts turned then to Bella Bella. I recalled the night when we had found the boardinghouse crowded with officials. Wally, weary from manipulating the pigeon through rain and fog, was soon sleeping soundly, his snores as startling as the rumbling of thunder. I'd never objected to these explosive sounds in the night, knowing that when they reached a certain volume, all was well with Wally. I'd close my eyes and join him in sleep.

Suddenly, that night, my eyes popped open. I sat bolt upright in bed. What was going on?

"Good God Almighty!" came a querulous voice. "Have you ever heard anything like it?"

Another voice exploded in profanity. Then the first voice took over. "Easy, man! There's a lady in there."

"Hell! No *lady* could sleep with that. Hit that damn wall again."

Well! They should be snoring, too. Then I heard Irene's small son cry and heard Irene stirring. The whole house was awake except for Wally, and I saw no reason to disturb him. He would simply fall back to sleep and continue to blast out.

Irene and I exchanged grins in the morning—a silent pact not to acquaint Wally with the night's happenings. He greeted each guest with a cheery "Good morning," and if their response was on the dour side, he dismissed it, reasoning that they would unbend with the first cup of coffee.

We liked Bella Bella, except for the rain and fog that plagued the area. If only there was something at Sullivan Bay! Many times we'd crept through fog and mist, fearful of missing that tiny haven, but always it was open, and we could depend on shelter. One night we found our cabin occupied by a group of young forestry men. Myrt certainly couldn't put the men out, nor would we have wanted her to. She solved the problem by scooting them over and hanging a curtain across one corner for us.

Our presence was acknowledged by a few nervous coughs, a few deep chuckles, and one voice intoning, "Uh-uh! No stories tonight." We undressed in the dark to avoid silhouettes.

We often found ourselves sharing that room, usually with an airline pilot. I'd wake in the morning not too surprised to see a hulking form in the bed across the room.

We liked these boys and their love of flying. Often, when the weather was marginal, they flew on ahead, then radioed back to Myrt, "Tell Doc Flynn it's okay."

Even with this relayed information, flying the coast was a hazardous business. We flew at altitudes ranging from fifty to six thousand feet and were not averse to sitting out a drifting fog patch. We flew when the skies were so blue the whole world shimmered. We flew when billowing cumulus clouds buffeted the pigeon and heavy rain limited visibility.

We risked our lives on almost every flight, yet it was an experience that neither of us wanted to give up. Flying was not easy or a lark. We were serious about our work, and about that wilderness home we both wanted. When we didn't find it, Wally looked for other interests.

Wally had begun to teach both Maureen and me to fly. Our pigeon had served us well, but it seemed she had outlived her usefulness. She could no longer carry all the supplies our expanding practice required. We had resorted to shipping part of the load, but delayed shipments made for confusion. We needed a larger plane. An Aeronca Sedan was given priority consideration, since it wouldn't be too great a change from the pigeon. Before we came to any decision, however, a friend, Fred Melberg, suggested an old Stinson SR5.

"They're becoming obsolete, Doc," he said. "But I flew one in the bush and it was a real workhorse. Darn sight sturdier than the newer planes. There's one hangared down south of Olympia. Why don't we have a look?"

It was twice the size of the pigeon, and Wally and Fred were impressed. She looked like a monster to me, and that's what I called her. The name remained, and though there was sadness in making the change, it was necessary.

A few days later Wally and Fred flew her to a small airstrip from which she could be transported to Kenmore for conversion to pontoons. There was much work to be done: wings recovered, a new paint job—our colors, of course, yellow and maroon. The new pontoons made the pontoons on the pigeon seem like toys.

At last she was ready to fly. Winds that had buffeted the pigeon had little effect on the monster. Wally had to show her off to Al, of course. Clowholm was our first test flight, and this time there was room for Maureen. That alone did more to reconcile me to the monster than any other feature.

Al's reception was all we'd hoped for. "What you flying, Doc? Thought for sure somebody important was coming in."

Civilization might catch up, but for the moment Clowholm was ours. During the weeks when our plane was being converted, Wally and Fred had spent countless evenings poring over maps. They were much alike, lovers of the out-of-doors, with an insatiable urge to seek out the unknown. Fred and his bride, Doris, were planning a boat trip up the Athabasca River in northern Alberta and along the hundred-mile stretch of Lake Athabasca in the Northwest Territories.

"Now there's a deal for you, Doc," Fred proposed. "For sure they won't have a veterinarian there. If you fly inland, after you finish your work at Prince Rupert, it would only be a matter of a thousand miles. How about it?"

A thousand miles! Three days' flying time at least. They spoke of it as casually as most people would of ten miles. I had studied Doris's quiet, gentle face. Did she really go along with these wild plans, or did she acquiesce because she was such a young wife? Whatever her feelings, she did leave with Fred, soon after our Clowholm flight. Engrossed in preparations for our Alaska flight, I forgot them. Until Wally began talking about Lake Athabasca.

"No!" I announced flatly. "I won't go."

I remembered only too well that long flight to New York: the heat, the turbulence, seaplane facilities marked on our maps but long closed and forgotten. Maps, I'd discovered,

didn't keep up with the times. I didn't like flying over great
stretches of land. I didn't like the worry of wondering if we
could make it from one water hole to another. I'd had enough
of that kind of flying.

Wally had looked at me in astonishment. I had at times
protested, but I had never uttered an unequivocal *no*, and *no*
it remained, in spite of Wally's protestations, until the day I
stopped in at the gas station owned by Fred's father.

"I guess you'll be seeing the kids on your trip up north,"
he said pleasantly.

"No," I replied. "We aren't planning on it."

"Oh!" He hesitated. "I was hoping you would. Doris is
pregnant. I'm worried about that little girl. I hoped maybe
you could fly her out."

It had been taken out of my hands. Of course we would go.

Chapter 19

A thousand miles to find Doris and we hadn't found her. I thought of the long trek from Prince Rupert, through the coastal mountains to the high plateau country of northern British Columbia, through the Rocky Mountain range and over the Peace River country. No veterinarians, Fred had said, and thus far, few people and no animals, either. At Fort McMurray, however, we'd gotten word of Doris and Fred. They were on the Athabasca River, heading back from Lake Athabasca.

The meandering Athabasca River cut a deep swath through the flat monotony of a country relieved only slightly by the now familiar growth of scrubby evergreens. Two hundred miles north of Fort McMurray and we were upon the lake. How could we have missed Doris and Fred? The intense heat of the day magnified my depression. To have come so far, only to fail.

"We won't give up," Wally affirmed as we headed back down the river. "They could have pulled into the bushes along the riverbank to get out of this beastly hot sun."

We flew low over the river, searching, searching. My eyes ached from the effort to probe those bushes. If they were in the bushes, why didn't they come out? They had to hear the roar of our engine, and Fred surely would recognize the Stinson.

And then I saw a scow ahead. Against our speed it seemed not to be moving at all. We circled back for a landing and pulled up alongside. I marveled at the amount of camping paraphernalia piled in that rather flat-bottomed boat. And I couldn't help but think, What a trip to take just to appease a pioneering instinct! Doris and Fred sat like statues, just staring, disbelieving. Then Fred found his voice.

"Doc! I should have recognized that plane when it flew over a while back, but I'd about given up looking for you."

I ached for Doris. She was heavy with child, and though she sat tall, there was a deep weariness in her eyes. The once fair skin had turned brown from months of exposure to the burning sun. Though I knew she was glad to see us, she barely smiled.

"We can't talk here," Fred said. "We'll meet you at Emberras, downriver. Can't be too far now."

Emberras was an airstrip built and maintained by Americans to service planes flying the DEW line, that three-thousand-mile network of radar stations north of the Arctic Circle. As we taxied up to the small river dock, I stood on the pontoon, rope in hand. Wally edged in closer, careful to avoid scraping our wing on the vertical red clay bank of the river. I saw men running down the trail to the dock. One of them untied an old rowboat and jumped in, his hand extended to assist me. I watched flabbergasted as, with hand still extended, he and the boat sank to the bottom of the river. Moments later he bobbed up, sputtering and spitting out water.

"Sure never expected to see a woman get out of that plane," he said. "Got so excited I forgot that damn boat had a leak and was half full of water."

Visitors were welcome, especially if one happened to be a woman. Eight young men lived here, only one of whom had a wife. She was pregnant. There was also a dog, a black female Labrador, and she was pregnant, too. I could understand the pregnancy in the woman, but was puzzled about the dog's condition. Settlements along the river were a hundred miles apart. A male would have to travel a long way.

"We flew in a male to keep her company for a while," one of the men explained. "Sure hope she'll be okay. She's our mascot."

I saw Wally's eyes light up. A thousand miles and he had found a patient. One or one hundred, it made no difference to him.

"Would you like me to check her over?" he asked. "I happen to be a veterinarian."

As he ran back to the plane for his bag, Jane, the young wife, came to meet me. She watched as Wally knelt on the ground beside the Lab.

"I hope my doctor is as concerned when my time comes," she said.

It was late when Doris and Fred arrived. One doesn't make much time with a 1½-horsepower inboard. It was too late to plan to fly on to Fort McMurray, even if Doris had been up to it. Exhausted, she went right to bed. The night's rest didn't help.

"We'll have to wait," I told Wally. "She isn't up to going anywhere yet."

"No hurry. That Lab's about to whelp. I'd like to be here."

In the afternoon Doris asked me to walk down to the dock with her. We were alone there. She lay down, flat on her back, her eyes squeezed shut. For a time I lay quietly at her side, but then I began to worry. She lay too still. She was quiet too long. I raised onto my elbow, studying her face. There was no tautness around the sensitive mouth, no furrows marring the smooth brow, but though her cheeks were dry, the dark lashes hiding her eyes were wet, and I knew she was crying.

Impulsively I leaned over and kissed her on the cheek. "Is it so awful, Doris?"

Her eyes opened and the tears spilled out. There was no outward cry, just that avalanche of tears. How long, I wondered, since she had permitted herself such an indulgence? At last she rolled over and, with an effort, sat up.

"I didn't mean to cry."

"I know."

"It's just . . . well . . . the thought of getting back in that boat. There's no room to move around. I get so tired just sitting, and the sun is down such a little while."

"We came here to fly you out, Doris. You don't have to get back in that boat."

Her eyes brightened, then clouded. "I don't know. We planned this together, Fred and I. I wanted to do it all the way."

"But now you both have someone else to think of," I reminded her.

It was decided we would leave, but the day was too hot to fly and the Lab hadn't whelped. Doris and Fred needed some time to talk things out. I didn't see much of Wally, but toward evening he came into Jane's house, his face aglow.

"As beautiful pups as I've ever seen. Nine of them!"

It was late evening when we took off for Fort McMurray. The monster climbed effortlessly to one thousand feet. Wally leveled out, and I glanced back to see how Doris was taking it. Her eyes were closed, but she had a quiet smile on her face.

Chapter 20

"Oh, I feel good!" Doris had joined us for a late breakfast in the same small café where we had first gotten word of her and Fred. "I'll walk to the dock with you when you're ready to leave. I could walk and walk and walk."

The shouts of laughter that reached our ears as we tramped down the road hardly prepared us for the hilarious scene at the dock. A group of youngsters, buckets brimming with river water, were fashioning a mud slide down the clay bank. Shoving, pushing, they slid into the water, headfirst, feet-first, sideways.

As Wally, dragging the long gas hose, climbed up onto the wing of the monster, my eyes strayed to the northeast horizon, where a peculiar funnel-shaped cloud was forming. Too small for a tornado, I decided, but I shouted to Wally anyway. He screwed the gas cap in place and jumped to the dock.

"Come on. Under the wing."

The funnel whipped over us. Rain and hail drummed against our fabric wing, making miniature whirlpools in the water. The children on the shore ran for the shelter of our wing. Those in the river swam between the pontoons and under the belly of the monster. In less than five minutes it was all over.

A small tornado, surely, but it had done no damage. The

kids, in fact, were delighted. They grabbed up handfuls of black mud and plastered each other from head to foot. Their slippery bodies looked like shiny black seals. Wally finished gassing the monster, and Doris and I walked with him to the flight shack.

Filing a flight plan is usually a simple procedure, but today our radio operator was having trouble. "Lot of static electricity in the air," he said. "If Peace River and Fort St. John can't hear me any better than I hear them, you haven't much of a flight plan."

Wally pulled at his lower lip with thumb and forefinger. "I don't much like flying around this country without a flight plan. Can you try it again?"

The operator nodded, then smiled at a young woman who walked in the door. She listened as he twisted the radio dials, repeating our message over and over: "Stinson N 14154 . . . Dr. Flynn . . . One passenger . . . Fort McMurray to Peace River . . . Time of arrival four P.M."

The young woman walked over to a large map stapled on the wall, then beckoned to me. "I'm Julie," she said. "My husband flies out of here. He's due in now." She frowned, then shrugged, accepting the unreliability of schedules. "I don't like the feel of the weather today. If it doesn't look good out there," and she made a vague motion, "head for Wabaska Lake." She pointed it out on the map. "There are two missions there. No one lives on any of the other lakes in the area."

"We only have maps for the route we'd mapped out," I told her. "Could we buy a map of that area here?"

"Sorry. We just get what we need out of Edmonton." She shrugged again. "Line Wabaska up with some lake on your map. In this country it pays to have an out."

I studied that map until I was certain every detail was etched in my mind. Then I heard the operator speak to Wally.

"I can't get weather, but I feel pretty certain of your flight plan. Made out their 'Roger' okay."

Wally was satisfied. Once again in the plane, we circled the dock. I could see Doris, looking up, waving. Wally dipped a wing in response, then headed west, back across that wooded expanse of no-man's-land. Maintaining altitude proved difficult. Heat from the tinder-dry bush pulled us earthward. It was unusual that, with such heat, there was no turbulence. We'd been out over an hour.

"It's so muggy," I observed. "I'm sticky all over."

"Yeah! I don't like it. Have you noticed that peculiar grayish tinge on the horizon? Could be haze, I suppose."

The gray deepened and spread, reaching out to encompass us. "Could it be a bush fire?" Wally wondered uneasily.

"It's a storm, I think. I've seen them like that in Montana."

"You could be right. Wonder if we could outrun it if we headed back to Fort McMurray?"

"I doubt it. Julie said to head for Wabaska. See that lake ahead? Wabaska is about sixty miles due south of it. It's the largest lake in the area, so I should recognize it."

Without a word, Wally wheeled about and headed south. I sat erect, searching the terrain, trying to recall every detail of that map on the wall. We realized this was no ordinary storm. The air was oppressive, and the mass in the sky, so near, was now a wicked black.

"There's the lake, Wally. The mission's at the far end." My voice pleaded, as though the pleading could, in some mysterious way, increase our speed. What if we didn't make it? Fear was like a phantom riding alongside us in the plane. My eyes were hot and dry, my throat felt parched, my tongue clung to the roof of my mouth, and my heart cried, "Faster! Faster!"

In the eerie stillness we seemed not to be flying at all, but rather to be suspended, sustained by an unseen force, as if the air were holding us prisoner. I could see the cluster of buildings, and the tiny dock extending out over the lake. Yet we couldn't set down. My hands knotted into fists. The lump in my throat threatened to choke me. What was the matter? What was holding us? Wally poured on the power, tearing us, at last, from the grip of that still air. There wasn't a ripple on the lake. Like the air, it appeared to be in the clutch of an inexplicable calm.

Suddenly we touched water, and I was out on the pontoon, looping my rope around the strut. The black mass was descending. I tossed the trailing end of the rope to a man who had waited for us. Then I leaped for the dock. Wally was right behind me as the ropes were hitched.

Then it was upon us. Day became night; the lake was swallowed by the blackness. Hurricane-force winds struck with a deafening howl, lashing the lake into monstrous waves that beat at our plane. She creaked and groaned, struggling to be free of the ropes that restrained her, lurching; one wing in the water, the other wing bashing the dock. Numb with horror, insensible to the wind and the rain and the hail, we watched her struggle.

"There she goes!" Wally's words were a sob.

She was over, one pontoon wedged under the dock, the other pontoon and the outside wing pointing skyward. My head throbbed with every frenzied beat of the inside wing against the dock.

"Leave her be! She's ours!" Was that my voice screaming defiance at the wind?

"God!" It was Wally. He dashed out and snatched at the wing, trying to hold it up off the dock.

Tearing myself free from arms that sought to restrain me, ignoring the warning I'd certainly be killed, I ran to join Wally. The dock threatened with every pitch to toss us into the seething waters, but we had become two wild creatures, devoid of self, possessed of a madness rivaling the demonic fury of the storm. We stubbornly clung to the tip of the wing, feeling no pain from bashed and bleeding fingers.

What possessed me to go farther? The dock was built in two sections, one section built out from the shore, another section across the end, forming a T. If I advanced to the point where the sections were joined, I reasoned, I could push up on the strut.

"Come back! Come back!" The words swept by me on the wings of the wind, and I paid them no heed.

As I took my stand on the precarious brink of the T, it sprang apart. My footing was gone. The relentless waves that had torn the dock now came thundering back, smashing the separated sections, one against the other. I felt the force of the waves and the weight of our four-thousand-pound plane as the broken dock seesawed the full length of my legs. Again the dock parted, and I was pulled free. But Wally was plunged into the churning waters. Other arms carried me to safety. Wally struggled to shore.

Wally put a hand on my arm. "We can't save her, Chicken." His voice was choked with emotion.

I had been content to be supported by the arms of the man who'd carried me to safety, but at Wally's words I made an effort to move. Then the pain came.

"I can't walk!"

"It's a miracle that your legs weren't severed." Paul Conrad, the Indian Agent, spoke up.

I endured the short ride in a truck to his home. The house was ablaze with lights. I suddenly became conscious of my muddy feet, and the water running in rivulets from my clothing.

"I can't come in," I wailed. "I'll ruin your floor."

"Never mind the floors. Please come in," Mrs. Conrad urged.

"No," I sobbed, giving way to hysteria. "I won't! I won't!"

Without a word, Wally carried me over the threshold and eased me into a chair. In the confusion of voices I heard Mrs. Conrad ask, "Is she badly hurt?"

She shook her head as she knelt to sponge warm water over my back. "I'm a nurse," she said. "I've seen my share of bruised bodies, but I've never seen the likes of you. We'll get you to bed."

Wally wasn't long in joining me, but our exhausted minds and bodies rejected sleep. Even the weight of the sheet was unbearable. I began to think of Betty King. Our decision to fly to the Athabasca country had angered her.

"You're a damn fool, Dr. Flynn," she had exploded. "Begging your pardon, Mrs. Flynn. But one man can't spread himself all over the north country. It's too damn big. You belong to Ketchikan. Together we make it a good place for animals to live. I let you go because you made a promise to your friends, but you come back in September, you hear?"

Chapter 21

"Why must it always happen to you?" Wally's voice shook as he lifted me from the bed the next morning and stood me on my feet. Could I walk? I forced my right leg forward, dragging the left into position. Mrs. Conrad heard us and came up the stairs.

"You're not out of bed!" she exclaimed.

Wally carried me downstairs and propped me up with pillows. While Mrs. Conrad prepared breakfast he stood at the window, staring out at the bleak skies, and I knew Betty King must be on his mind, too.

"Is there some way we can get out of here?" he asked abruptly.

"If you're thinking of towing your plane out," she replied, "it's ninety miles to Lesser Slave. That's our nearest settlement. There's a road, but this is muskeg country. The road's usable only in the winter, when the ground is hard frozen."

"My God!" Wally interrupted. "This is only July."

"Well, there's a small airstrip across the point at Desmarais, the Catholic mission. A plane should be there in a couple of weeks maybe. You could go and come back for your plane." She didn't add, If it is worth coming back for. But what would we be without our plane?

I watched through the window as Wally strode down the road to the dock. His cap was pulled low over his eyes, and his shoulders were hunched against the wind and the rain.

"Took an awful beating," he said as he came back in the door, "but she's all in one piece. We can patch her up and she'll be as good as new."

We turned on the radio for word of the storm, a hurricane, which had swept on over the Fort McMurray area. And then: "Reported missing on a flight to Peace River, Dr. Flynn and one passenger."

I sucked in my breath. What fears they could conjure up in the minds of loved ones who heard them! It was only a local report from Peace River that we'd heard. Before that report went farther, surely we'd get a message to Maureen. And what of Doris and Fred? Doris should have been safe at the hotel, but what of Fred, putting down the river with his 1½-horsepower inboard?

Wally paced the floor. "They'll start a search once this storm's blown itself out. We can't have that. It costs too much and it endangers too many others. We've got to get a message out, let them know we're safe."

"They have a radio transmitter at Desmarais," Mrs. Conrad said. "Maybe Father Fillion can get a message out. Paul's coming up the walk now. He can take you over."

When Wally and Paul returned I knew at once they'd had no luck. Atmospheric conditions had interfered with transmission, Wally told me, but Father Fillion had promised to keep trying.

He kept his promise, trudging the muddy mile across the point innumerable times, just to reassure us. We came to look forward to his double rap at the door and his cheery "Hello there! And how are we doing?"

On the morning of the fourth day Father Fillion burst into the kitchen, barely pausing to knock. "Made it! Got your messages out. Even got an answer."

He'd canceled our flight plan and had notified Maureen that we were safe. Two men would be flown in from Edmonton in the morning, to work on the monster.

The plane from Edmonton roared overhead early the next

morning, and soon Father Fillion arrived at the Conrads' with two tall young men in tow, Jim Godden and Al Johnson. Father Fillion turned to me.

"The plane's waiting to take you to the hospital."

Accusingly, I turned to Wally. "You never told me."

"I know, Chicken, but you're so damned obstinate. I figured if the plane came and you knew you were expected . . ."

I didn't care that my legs barely functioned. Wally and I were in this together.

A cursory examination of the monster revealed holes in the fuselage and in the tail section. One wing tip was shattered, and there was that gaping hole in the pontoon.

Al shook his head. "If we get this bird flying, we'll really rate our tickets."

Al underestimated the ingenuity of the mission people. Mr. Tarran took a copper rod from a discarded refrigerator. It gave form to the wing. For the stays, Mr. Godwin, the Anglican minister, donated excess stripping that had been purchased for the church pews. The women of both the Anglican and Catholic missions cut and sewed sheets to cover the damaged wing tip.

The repair of the pontoon had been left for last. For this job the plane had to be entirely out of the water. With a rope tied to a rod inserted through holes in the pontoons and into cart wheels, then to the back of Paul's truck, our plane was pulled from the lake. Battered and torn, she had become our pigeon. The wheels and the rod were removed, and she sat firmly on solid ground.

Al and Jim studied the hole in the pontoon. The aluminum patching they'd brought would have to be bolted on, requiring the cooperation of two men, one working from inside the pontoon. Those pontoons had seemed so huge—twenty feet long, three feet deep, and three feet wide at the bottom, tapering up to one and a half feet across the top. One after another, the men attempted to squirm through the ten-by-eighteen-inch opening on the top of the pontoon. It was hopeless— they simply didn't fit.

There was no denying that unless I could slide into that compartment, the pigeon would have to wait for the winter freeze. What would Betty King think, and Lucy? The men lifted me up and lowered me through the opening, yet they couldn't assist me into position. Taking the pillows Wally had pulled from the plane, I laid them behind me. Then, flat on my back, I inched toward that hole. For a moment I lay panic-stricken. It was so dark in there, and there was a rank, musty odor. I inched on back to the hole and stuck my hand through as a sign of reassurance.

For nearly an hour I lay in that cramped position, keeping the nuts in place until each bolt held. Finally a shout came from outside. "It's finished." My arms fell to my sides.

"Okay in there?"

Anxious eyes peered through the opening. Voices shouted encouragement. Could I move? Every muscle protested as I edged forward.

"Come on, Muscles!" It was Wally's voice. "You can do it."

I inched forward again, Wally's voice egging me on, and as my head appeared through the opening a cheer went up. Wally lifted me from the pontoon and carried me up onto the bank.

"We're crazy!" His voice held a question. "You shouldn't have gone in there. I shouldn't have let you. What's with us?"

"It's not just us. It's her, the pigeon. She's us, sorta. It's all the people here. They've worked so hard. And everyone in Prince Rupert and Ketchikan expecting us in September. Some things you have to do."

"I know!" He laid his big hand over mine. "This will set us back a few years, Chicken. Labor like this doesn't come cheap. And that pontoon, even with the patch, is no damn good. We'll have to get a new pontoon in Edmonton before we can go on home."

He leaned over and kissed my forehead with just the brush of his lips.

Chapter 22

Our pigeon was back in the water. Our friends had gathered to wish us Godspeed on our flight to Edmonton. Ahead of us lay 180 miles, which, again, we must navigate without the benefit of maps. We had studied the area map on the mission wall, and I had drawn a sketch of sorts. Would our pigeon, with her makeshift patches, perform under pressure?

Amid shouts of optimism, we taxied out from the dock. Wally poured on the power. There was speed, but no lift. Our injured wing sagged, and we knew the damaged pontoon was taking on water.

Twice we were forced to return to the dock. We removed our baggage, and then the back seat—anything to lighten the load.

For the third time we taxied out. Our pigeon wobbled, half lifted, and sank back. Wally's mouth tightened.

"I'll pull her off on one pontoon. There's no other way."

He pulled hard to the right, and the damaged pontoon shot out of the water. Giving her full power, we sped along on that one good pontoon until, unbelievably, we were free. Water trailed from the leaky pontoon. I felt the flutter of our patched wing and shivered in turn, but the pigeon climbed steadily. A dip, a quiver, and we were on our way.

We could hardly mistake seventy-mile-long Lesser Slave Lake, but from there on innumerable small lakes were difficult to identify with only my sketch for verification. Increas-

ingly heavy cloud conditions blotted out a lake or a town
I had so carefully marked. Leaving the lake country, we flew
over rolling farmland with tiny villages tucked between the
hills, glimpsed briefly between cloud patches. I searched for
a clue that we were on course. Wally was intent on a more
promising solution, his fingers twisting the radio dial. If he
could locate Edmonton radio, we could beam in.

"Hey! I've got it." And he held the phone to my ear so
that I, too, could hear the reassuring beep.

Seven miles to the south of Edmonton, briefly revealed by
the shifting clouds, lay Cooking Lake. We were met at the
ramp by a few men, one of whom drove us to a hotel in Edmonton.

We were a week in Edmonton, waiting for the installation
of the new pontoon. During the week the cut in my thigh
firmed and the greenish color faded.

The best news was that Fred was safe. He'd been picked up
by one of the stern-wheelers that carry freight up the river.
They'd pulled in to a high bank and the storm had swooshed
over their heads, ripping out trees and anything that stood
in its way. Fred had met Doris in Fort McMurray and they
were on their way back to Seattle by train.

And now we were going home, too. We flew to Wabaska
to pick up our bags, then backtracked to the village of Lesser
Slave to replenish our fuel and to stay the night. On this
particular day, crews engaged in the search for oil were
changing shifts, and the one hotel, a two-story frame building,
was jammed. Cigarette smoke permeated the vestibule, and
the din of voices pounded in my ears. I walked outside and
sat on the high curbing. I doubted the hotel had even twenty
rooms. The fact that I was a woman, the only woman, would
make no difference. I wondered if the men resented me.

With nothing else to do, I studied them. The replacement
crew was cleanshaven, a restless group, determined to enjoy to
the hilt whatever entertainment the town could offer. The
outgoing crew was bearded, dirty, weary, wanting only to
sleep. They were all young men. One came to sit beside me
on the curb.

"It's hell out there," he said. "Ten days of pure hell!"

"Is that as long as you stay out?"

"Any longer would kill a man. We grow these damn beards and wear nets over our heads, but even so the mosquitoes and the black flies make mincemeat of us. And nothing can keep out the no-see-ums." He was silent a moment, running grubby fingers through his beard.

"Whole damn country's muskeg. Treacherous stuff, that muskeg, worse than quicksand. Water fills into hollows. Moss grows in and then the brush. Can't tell till you hit it whether the ground's solid or not. Our machines travel in pairs. It's nothing to see the front machine sink clear in. We haul it out and search for a spot where maybe we can get through. A man has to want money damn bad. Hell! It ain't worth it."

Someone called to him. There was a room, and he hurried to claim it. I sat wondering how we would have fared the day of the storm if we hadn't made it to Wabaska. Except for the fact that there were no settlements on that four-hundred-mile stretch from Fort McMurray to Peace River, the country had not looked too fearsome. In fact, the many lakes had given me a false sense of security. Mrs. Conrad had mentioned that the road was built over muskeg. It had not occurred to me that in many places that muskeg would not bear even the weight of a body.

Then Wally obtained a room. The clerk thrust another key into my hand.

"The toilet's at the end of the hall, ma'am. This is the only key."

Behind the closed door, I turned to Wally in panic. "If I have to walk down that hall, you walk with me. I won't walk alone."

"Nobody's going to bother you."

"What if somebody wants my key?"

"Nobody will; it's a big outdoors."

Our course led us in a northwesterly direction to Charlie Lake the next day. Another storm delayed us there, but when patches of blue showed through the gray we sneaked through Pine Pass in the Rockies, heading for the Coast Range and the salt waters we knew so well.

"There's a shortcut through the Coast Range. Let's try it."

As we entered the narrow, twisted gorge, the clouds closed in, giving us only distorted glimpses of the route we must follow. Many times, during periods of stress, my stomach had churned, but it had never actually jumped up and down as it was doing now.

Wally shook his head. "Okay, Chicken, where do you want to go through?"

"Let's take the Bella Coola Valley. According to the map, it's a straight cut through the mountains. And people live there!" This had suddenly become very important.

In this sea-level valley, hemmed in by ten-thousand-foot peaks, little farms were laid out as methodically as patchwork. At the western exit the town of Bella Coola hugged the shore of Burke Channel. A fog bank at water level was moving rapidly up the channel. We dived, gaining access to the water just as the fog swept over the town, blanking it out so completely I almost doubted I'd actually seen it.

Sullivan Bay was around the bend and down just a stretch. Bruce met us at the float with news.

"We've decided to have a go at logging, Doc. Sullivan's up for sale. How about it?"

Wally's eyes lit up. How long we'd waited and searched for someplace like this. Now it was offered. But then he shook his head. "Gad! It's a temptation. But, no! Running this place is a full-time job. I've seen that. It would mean no more flying, no more veterinary medicine."

Chapter 23

"You've got to come to Sitka, Dr. Flynn." Jerry O'Connell leaned forward, pushing a mop of carrot-red hair from her face. "Why can't you?"

"I see dinner's ready. Let's discuss it while we have some of that meat you girls were clamoring for," Wally suggested.

When asked what they'd like for dinner, both Maureen and Jerry had said, "*Meat*," a change from the starchy diet served at the dormitory where they had been assigned a room together when both had entered Seattle University in September.

Jerry, with her fondness for animals, had fit into our anomalous household. That fondness led naturally to the question she had posed before dinner.

"So you think we should come to Sitka?" Wally asked her now. "You realize there's more to it than just going? We'd need advance advertising and a place to work."

Jerry pushed back from the table, scooping Gardenia up from the floor. "If that's all, you're as good as there. I'll make all the arrangements. You won't have a worry. Okay?"

"Seems to be settled," Wally agreed.

She jumped to her feet, inadvertently dislodging Gardenia, who, shrilling in protest, stomped to Wally's chair, digging her nails into the upholstery as she attempted to pull herself up.

"There, old girl!" He bent over and picked her up. "Not quite so easy anymore, is it?"

"Oh, Gardenia, I'm sorry. Please come back," Jerry pleaded. But Gardenia turned baleful eyes, hissing her defiance.

"Never mind, Jerry. Another half hour she'll be demanding to sit in your lap."

A day or so later Wally charged into the kitchen waving a letter. From Fred.

Fred and Doris, after returning to Seattle, stayed just long enough for a tiny son to make his appearance. Then Fred had found property on Vancouver Island near the village of Tofino and had moved his family to the island. We hadn't met the new addition to the family, for, true to our word, and in spite of makeshift repairs on our pigeon, we had flown back to the north country to carry on with our September clinics.

"Fred wants us to come up," Wally announced now. "Says we might like a chunk of his land."

"Now?" I protested. "In January? It's snowing, and anyway, the pigeon isn't ready to fly."

"I know. More work than I anticipated replacing all those patches. We could drive to Port Alberni and take a local flight out, though."

"Seems silly, this time of the year, and not even a road out." I glanced up, saw the disappointment in his eyes. Reaching over, I rumpled his hair. "Let's go!"

Snow spewed from the spinning prop of the plane as we flew down the Alberni Canal, but I did not regret my decision. The inaccessibility of the island's west coast was a challenge. I liked its mountain ruggedness, and as we tramped through the snow with Doris and Fred, I sensed their contentment. Still, we left with no commitments made for our own plans to settle down.

The demands of the hospital and plans for our work in the North, which now included Sitka, drove thoughts of Tofino from our minds. Jerry left for Sitka in early June, and we soon followed.

Lilliputian islands jutted from the sea, forming a protective harbor for the town. About half the size of Ketchikan, it sprawled at the foot of a snowcapped mountain. Jerry had recognized our plane as we circled the town and was waiting for us at the dock.

"You made it!"

As she drove she pointed out Pioneer Home, where old-time Alaskans came to spend their last years. Two blocks from the dock the street split to encircle a church. It was grayed and weather-beaten, but distinctive in its styling, with a rounded dome and a bell tower. It was evident that the church had been there first and the town had sprung up around it. Jerry slammed to a stop.

"That's St. Michael's, our old Russian church. I'll take you in. Mom won't have lunch ready for a while anyway."

We were hardly prepared for the magnificence inside, the gold and silver icons, the rich velvets, the jeweled crowns. There was a peace that demanded silence.

"See that building across the street?" Jerry asked when we were outside. "That's where you'll be working. I have some appointments all set up for you . . . tomorrow."

After lunch we inspected our work quarters. Jerry had left nothing to chance. Wally was delighted with the hand-drawn signs in the windows and on the door of our newest clinic. We had a feeling that if clients didn't appear of their own volition, Jerry would haul them in.

Sitka had the same problem that characterized all southeastern Alaska towns, an overpopulation of animals. We had the usual spays and castrations. We had the usual complaints: decayed teeth, pussy ears, skin irritations. We also had four boxers with ears to be cropped. Usually ears are cropped when the animal is just a few months old. These were adult boxers. Still, the ears stood nicely. Then an Irish setter was brought in with a mangled front leg.

"Kids race their cars along the beach road," the setter's owner told us. "I've tried to break Clancy of chasing cars, but he just will run. This time he got it."

"He certainly did," Wally agreed. "I'm sorry, but that leg can't be saved. We'll have to amputate."

Horror spread over the man's face. "What good's a three-legged dog?"

"Do you use him for hunting?" Wally asked.

"No, he's just a pet, but a damn good one, in spite of his bad habits."

"He'll still be a good one. There won't be an ugly stump showing. We'll take it off right at the chest. The hair will soon cover the scar, and you'll find he'll run as good as ever. I would suggest, though, if he starts chasing cars again, that you let a long chain dangle around his neck. It won't hurt him, but it will be an annoyance and will slow him down."

Though she didn't say so, we suspected the real reason Jerry had been so determined to get us to Sitka was the welfare of a pair of bloodhounds.

The entire town of Sitka claimed these hounds, and rightly so. They had pooled their money to buy the dogs for rescue work. Many times hunters and hikers had become lost in the jagged mountains that made up the most of Baranof Island. These dogs had proven themselves as saviors with their highly developed sense of smell. Small wonder these dogs were the pride of Sitka.

The work in Sitka, combined with a heavy schedule in Ketchikan and Prince Rupert, kept us in the North until mid-July. It was good to be home again, back with Vicki and Minx and Spif and Gardenia. Most of all, I was glad to be with Maureen. Our times together, snatched from separate routines, were precious. But Seattle could hold Wally only so long.

"We promised Doris and Fred we'd take another look at their place this summer," he reminded me.

"I know, but somehow, after seeing Sitka . . ."

"Yeah! Well, maybe we'll feel differently when we get to Fred's."

Fred's property faced on a thirty-mile stretch of road that linked Tofino with the neighboring village of Ucluelet. Although that was the extent of the road, the prospect of even that many cars whizzing past our door was disturbing to Wally.

"Give us a few days to think it over, Fred. We'll head up to Muchalot Lake. I think better when I'm fishing."

While we were refueling at the dock in Tofino, a young missionary priest wandered down and stood watching us.

"Beautiful day," he said.

"Yes, isn't it?"

And so, quite naturally, we spoke of our wish for a home somewhere in this land of sea and mountains.

"Well now," the young priest said thoughtfully. "I know a place. Two English ladies own it. One's a teacher, but she's reached retirement age. The other's in her seventies. Really too isolated a spot for either of them. Let me see your map."

With a pencil he indicated a tiny cove about two-thirds of the way up the west coast of Vancouver Island, on the northwest tip of Nootka Island. Since we were flying north anyway, it wouldn't take us far out of our way.

"Just tell them Father Lobsinger sent you," the young priest suggested as we climbed aboard the pigeon.

Could that cove be the elusive home we had been searching for? The priest's arrival at the dock, coinciding as it did with our departure, seemed somehow prophetic.

North of Tofino, we found no roads. It was a majestic yet forbidding landscape, with forested mountains rising abruptly from the sea and a series of rocky reefs, pounded by angry breakers, dotting the coastline. And then, there we were, circling the cove.

A string of tiny islands was centered in the cove, restraining the rougher waters of Esperanza Inlet. Back from the cove rose five-hundred-foot Newton Hill, and beyond this hill and at the foot of towering Mount Rosa lay Owasitsa Lake. The property, as Father Lobsinger had described it, extended from the salt water of the inlet to the fresh water of the lake. The blue of the inlet blended into the green waters of the cove, the deep green of the forest merged into the deeper blue of Owasitsa Lake, and beyond stretched the subdued gray-blue of the Pacific. We could see two houses, one at the water's edge on the west bank of the cove, the other on a bluff, directly opposite, almost hidden in the trees.

We swooped low, studying our landing area. Ragged reefs, barely discernible below the water's surface, formed a natural barrier, transforming this peaceful cove into an impregnable fortress, advantageous, perhaps, to those within the barrier, but a decided hazard to one who would enter.

Exaggerated gestures from below directed us to a rocky spot on the west beach near the picturesque little house we hoped was for sale. It was quaintly English, tucked in amid the trees, with an unobstructed view of sea and mountains.

I was now aware of greetings. Both little ladies talked simultaneously.

"Father Lobsinger sent you, you say? Now wasn't that nice of him! No, it's not for sale"—indicating the little cottage that so entranced me—"but you must see ours."

Chattering away, they led us around the cove and up a bluff to an old log house. In comparison with the charming cottage across the cove it seemed stark and ugly, and I wondered if the sun ever found its way in, for the house was smothered by the advancing forest.

The gloom did not affect our hostesses. "Come in! Come in!" they chirped, opening a door and darting in ahead of us.

The kitchen, extending the full length of the house, was painted an off-brown and was sternly furnished in the same depressing shade. The storage cupboards and the table were handmade. There was a wood stove and, one concession to the times, a sink. But there were no faucets, no water inlets or outlets.

The living room was more appealing, its log walls grayed, the ceiling beams gleaming a rich mahogany. There was a room on either side, one of which had served as a chapel for the Indians. It had been left intact, as if just waiting for the proper time to come again. A stairway in the living room led to three sunnier rooms. These rooms, with their high cedar paneling and secret closets, so delighted me I could have ignored the kitchen, which apparently was nothing more than an afterthought tacked onto the original log building. Across the front of the building these unpredictable ladies had built on another lean-to, an enclosed porch that effectively shut out any light that might have trickled through the trees. Down on the beach was another building in a decrepit state.

"First post office in this area!" they announced proudly. "The Newtons started all this when the island was opened to homesteading. Most people couldn't make a go of it. Still pretty wild, cougar even. You do shoot, don't you?"

"I think we can take care of ourselves," Wally assured them.

They had admitted the worst. Now they almost pounced in their eagerness. "You do like it?"

As Wally turned to me, I raised an eyebrow ever so slightly. "We like it," he said, "but we'll have to talk it over. We'll let you know."

"Oh!" Their disappointment spilled out. "But don't wait too long. We must sell."

"We'll let you know as soon as we can, but now we must go."

"Oh, but you can't go. We haven't served tea. We always serve tea when we have company."

Over tea we learned more about these two little ladies. Miss Langdale, the teacher, was quite satisfied with her spinster status. Men always died off when you needed them the most anyway, she asserted. Take poor Mrs. Ball. Husband dead some ten years now. She was so alone. Naturally Miss Langdale had felt compassion for her, had invited her to live with her. Miss Langdale did most of the talking. Mrs. Ball appeared not to mind, smiling gently, nodding in agreement.

"Actually, it is I who own the property," Miss Langdale went on. "No one pays any attention to that, of course. Most everyone thinks we own it together. You see, I really need someone to look after the house when I'm away teaching, only, of course, now I'm not teaching anymore. Sixty-five, you retire, no matter how many good years you have left."

It was hard to break in, but Wally managed. "Where did you teach?"

"At Kyuquot. I taught the Indian children there. It's about thirty miles north of here. I went by boat. Generally Father Lobsinger took me. I came home weekends, unless the weather was too bad. Sometimes I was there two, three weeks at a time."

I looked at Mrs. Ball. Poor Mrs. Ball. So alone, Miss Langdale had said. Yet here she sat in this wilderness cove two and three weeks at a time, completely alone. It was hard to justify Miss Langdale's reasoning, but Mrs. Ball's serenity seemed to verify that, whatever the reasoning, she had accepted it. I wondered now who was the more anxious to leave.

"Mrs. Ball makes out fine," Miss Langdale continued. "Slim Beale, he lives in Zeballos, he comes out once a week or so and brings in supplies."

Miss Langdale was still talking when we got into the pigeon and waved good-bye. The last words we heard were, again, "Don't you wait too long now."

As we taxied out I took another good look at the cottage. Miss Langdale had maintained an indifference toward it. Any questions we'd managed to ask had been pushed aside. She would not reveal who owned the cottage, and had said it was not for sale.

It was but an hour's flight to Muchalot and still early enough for a bit of fishing. Later, as we relaxed in a cabin, I couldn't refrain from comparing it with the old log house at the cove. This cabin was bright and cheery, with a large picture window looking out over the lake. The opposite wall was dominated by a large stone fireplace, radiating its heat to the farthest corners. We had used the wood that had been stacked at the back door. Before we left we would cut more wood, replenish the supply of canned foods in the kitchen with cans of our own, and sign the guest book as others before us had done.

We awoke the next morning to the clatter of rain on the roof, and noted that the pass to the lake was completely obscured. Where else could one be more pleasantly marooned? Our thoughts wandered back to that house at the cove.

"If I didn't keep ending up in that awful kitchen," I complained.

"Well, would you rather build at Fred's?"

"Not after seeing the cove. Give me a little time. Maybe I'll get used to the idea of that kitchen."

There was another trip to Alaska, and still I hesitated.

November brought an urgent letter from our ladies, who had closed up the house and moved to Vancouver. If we wanted the property, they wanted an immediate reply. Another letter followed in December. We were almost persuaded when Christmas activities interfered, and in January we made a rush trip to Los Angeles to attend a veterinary symposium. The letter and the cove were forgotten.

Before we left Los Angeles, at the conclusion of the symposium, we visited with my sister and brother-in-law, Berne and Jack Hamilton. Somehow the conversation worked around to a discussion of the cove.

"Man!" Jack exclaimed. "You couldn't buy a lot in town for the price they quoted you. I'd grab it."

Suddenly it became very important to me to own the cove, including the house and that awful kitchen.

"What if they've sold to someone else!"

"Your mind's made up then?" Wally's eyes were twinkling.

"It is. I'll write them a letter the minute we get home."

On March 11, 1957, we met them in Vancouver. Miss Langdale was quite severe. "You almost waited too long. We were about to sell to someone else." But she melted into smiles when we signed the papers that made us the proud owners of a delightful cove, an old log house, and 112 acres of timber in the rugged wilderness of Nootka Island.

Chapter 24

The ramp man at Kenmore Air Harbor shook his head as he surveyed the back seat of our pigeon. It was stacked to the ceiling with food, clothing, all the essentials of housekeeping, and an ax, a saw, and other assorted tools.

"You guys have got to be out of your minds. What's so great about living in the bush anyway?" he demanded. "No roads, no neighbors. And in April? You could at least have waited for decent weather."

We couldn't wait. Three hours' flying time separated us from all that was old and familiar and thrust us, irrevocably, into a challenging new life. As we circled the cove I twisted in my seat, craning to see. It was all ours! Wally swooped down for a landing, then leaned over to pop a kiss on the tip of my ear.

"Cut the nonsense," I protested. "We're running out of water."

We'd never given it a thought that a good part of the water in our cove might go out with the tide. We didn't even own a book on the tides. One hadn't been necessary on our trips north, since floating ramps could adjust. Here there was no ramp. We must learn to deal with the tide. Slipping a rope over the pontoon cleats, front and back, we waded to shore, looping our ropes over a boulder.

We rounded the cove and climbed the steps up the bluff. This was *our* house.

The house was as brown and as dreary as I'd remembered it, only now it was damp and musty besides. Mold lay thick on the humble furnishings. The stove was rusted from months of disuse. The greatest shock came with the realization that the house had not long remained unoccupied. When the little ladies had moved out, the rats and mice had moved in. It was ghastly. We stood there, irresolute, uncertain, and suddenly it was funny. We rocked with laughter and the tears rolled down our cheeks and still we laughed.

"No picnic!" Wally gasped when we had regained a semblance of sobriety.

"No picnic," I agreed, laughter still choking my voice.

"A cup of coffee might help, though," Wally suggested. "I'll get our Thermos from the pigeon."

The respite was brief. If we hoped to sleep here this night, much had to be done. Wally chopped wood and built a fire to take the chill from the house. I scrounged a bucket from the pigeon and carried water from the creek to heat on the stove. We scrubbed . . . the table, the chairs, every piece of furniture there was. We swept and we mopped, and were utterly weary, but the house was warm and the clean smell of disinfectants had supplanted the mustiness. With a sort of dogged satisfaction, we surveyed our home, though pretty it was not.

"Don't worry," Wally assured me. "We'll paint it."

Though we welcomed night with its promise of sleep, there was a persistent scuttling of tiny feet as those miserable creatures who shared our home scurried about their business of finding food, building nests, or whatever. Their activities never ceased until the first rays of the sun peeked in our bedroom window. As if on signal, the night noises came to a halt. I snuggled down for a long-overdue sleep.

In the light of a new day our situation didn't seem so formidable. There was an indefinable charm about the old house that no amount of brown paint could efface. We wandered through the rooms, seeing the possibilities, noting the changes we'd make.

"There's one change we can't put off," Wally declared. "Just let me get my clippers working on that damn brush. You'll see some magic in here. Want to help me haul the stuff away?"

It was hard work, and I was the first to call it quits. "My aching back!" I protested. Wally tossed the clippers aside. "Okay. Let's call a halt. Lunchtime anyway."

"Hey!" I exclaimed as we opened the door. "It *is* magic. I can even see in the corners."

"How about that! I believe we're going to like it here."

"Except for one thing. The mice are bad enough, but those rats! They drive me up the wall."

"We certainly can't have that," Wally said, and he went out to poke around in the woodshed. In a few minutes he returned dragging a wicked-looking steel contraption. "An old muskrat trap, I think," he said. "It ought to do the trick."

Who would believe we could actually enjoy packing water from a stream, chopping wood, cooking over a rusty stove, and eating dinner by the light of a kerosene lamp? But if no one believed, did it even matter?

"Let's have a look at the old post office," Wally suggested. "Can't just sit here on the rocks all day."

Poking around, we found a slot marked MAIL, and along one wall were individual boxes. We picked up old ledgers the Newtons had kept and thumbed through them. So this had been a store as well!

"Center Island," Wally observed. "That's what they called this place. You know something, I think we got us a town after all—a ghost town, of course."

I giggled. "Do you suppose the ghosts are still about?"

"I'm serious. There's a lot of history here. Sometime I'm going to find out more about it."

"Okay, but let's change the name. 'Flynn's Cove' sounds better."

"You're staying then?"

"You know it."

Our preparations for bed that night included setting up that awful steel trap. It did give me a feeling of security.

Despite the scurrying feet, I fell asleep. The night was pitch-black when I sat up with a start. Ghosts? There was a most dreadful clanging, punctuated by shrill screams. I sat shivering, too terrified to move. Then I knew. The trap! Some unwary rat must have tripped the trigger and sprung those cruel jaws. But did he have to drag it all over the house, screaming at every step? Why couldn't he just die? Wally snored peacefully beside me.

Reaching for my flashlight, I searched the room for a weapon. The beam of my light picked out an old broom handle. With the flashlight in one hand and the broom handle in the other, I crept down the stairs. The rat screamed again. Holding my light on the hapless creature, I struck, again and again, until the awful screams were silenced. Trembling, I sank back against the wall. Though it seemed more merciful to kill the wretch than to let him scream in agony all night, I was repelled by the portentousness of my deed. Turning away, I climbed the stairs.

The sun was streaming through the window when next I awoke. I could hear Wally stirring around in the kitchen, but it was pleasant in bed and I made but a halfhearted motion to rise. It was enough. Wally bounded up the stairs bearing a tray.

"Breakfast, my lady!" He looked as pleased as a cat with a saucer of cream. "Guess what? We caught a rat in our trap. Odd, though! He was only caught by a foot. One would think he'd chew himself free. That's the nature of the animal. All I can figure is his shock reserve was low and he died of shock."

"Shock my eye!" I retorted. "I beat him to death."

"You what?"

"I beat him to death," I repeated, relating the night's happenings, "and you just kept on snoring."

"Well! That certainly shoots my theory all to hell." Then he began to laugh, and the laugh became a roar. "Sometimes I think I don't know you at all."

Fortunately for my peace of mind, the rats were soon either exterminated or discouraged. Then the ranks of mice filled in faster than we could deplete them. I'd gasp involuntarily when a particularly bold one darted across the floor.

There were delights, however, that more than compensated for our unending battle with the mice. There were walks through the forest and along the beach, and hours sitting in the sun, daydreaming. We learned to relax to a degree we would never have believed possible.

"Are we ever the procrastinators," Wally reflected one sunny afternoon. "We should fly to Zeballos and restock on food. It's only fourteen miles, but darned if I feel like going."

"Let's not. I'm not hungry."

"That's a switch. But you will be. Say, there's a speedboat. Wonder where it's going!"

We waved, and to our surprise, the boat turned and headed into the cove. Barney Howard, from the Indian village of Nuchatlitz, four miles southwest of us around the curve of the island, was our neighbor.

"You want something?" Barney's greeting caught us off guard. Wally fumbled for an answer.

"We didn't think you'd see us. We didn't think anyone knew we were here."

"We know. We see the plane other times when we go by. You want something?" he persisted.

Wally hesitated only a moment. "As a matter of fact, we were talking of flying to Zeballos for groceries."

"You tell me what you want. I'll buy for you."

He seemed so eager. And what a break for us. But he didn't continue on toward Zeballos. Instead, he turned and headed across the inlet, in the direction of Queens Cove, where, we knew from our map, there was a fish camp and store. He was making a special trip just for us.

April 17 arrived, a stormy, rainy Easter Sunday. We were up early, teasing each other with impossible hiding places for the eggs we had boiled and decorated with pen and ink the day before. Our hunt was interrupted by the whine of an engine.

"That boat's coming in here," I cried.

The boat, a fishing troller, approached to within hailing

distance. "Father Lobsinger say come to Mass," the Indian at the helm announced gravely. So the young priest was again directing our destiny. On the way to Nuchatlitz we learned the name of our pilot: Alban Michael, son of Chief Felix Michael.

After Mass we walked with Father Lobsinger to the home of Alban and his wife, Rose. We met Chief Felix, and Barney again, and many others. No one knocked, but they came, in one door, out another, on the opposite sides of the room.

Rose had prepared an Easter breakfast of hard-boiled eggs, homemade bread and jam, and coffee. The men, those who were invited, gathered at a table set in the middle of the room. Rose motioned to me to join them. On benches around the room women sat with children on their laps, others clinging to their knees, silent, watchful. Occasionally one of the women would get up and herd her charges out the door. Her place was not left vacant.

Wally laughed and joked with the men, but I fit in neither with the amiable group at the table nor with the women. I squirmed under the intensity of their gaze, the eggs and bread lumped in my throat. Would the meal never end? But at last! Chairs scraped as the men rose and filed through the door. The women and children followed. Rose and I were alone, and I was more uncomfortable than ever. What did one say to an Indian woman? There seemed no mutual interest on which to base a conversation.

"Could I help you with the dishes?" I managed at last.

"Yes," she replied, handing me a towel.

As we set to work, she began to speak. Her voice was musical, and so soft I had to strain to hear. The lovely features of her round face were enhanced by the velvety brown of her eyes. Long black hair swung freely about her shoulders. My uneasiness vanished, and in our eagerness to know each other, the words tumbled out.

Wally and I ventured out from our cave only when dwindling supplies necessitated a trip to Queens Cove. Father Lobsinger stopped in on his trips back and forth, often staying to dinner. We came to know the sound of his boat and would dash to the beach to welcome him as he maneuvered past our reefs. We came to depend on this young man with the ready smile and the sparkle in his blue eyes. A problem, to us insurmountable, with his help became no problem at all. Stovepipes to be cleaned. Repairs that could not wait. Running his fingers through curly brown hair, he invariably came up with the same stock answer.

"Well, let's have at it."

We couldn't indefinitely separate ourselves from Seattle, for the hospital was still our responsibility. We timed our return to coincide with Maureen's birthday, May 27. Now we would have the opportunity to see Zeballos, since the pigeon must be serviced before the flight back.

Leaving our pigeon at the ramp, we strolled up the single dusty street, past the post office, a machine shop, the general store, a café, a small hotel, a bakery, and a scattering of houses. It was pleasant wandering down the street, nodding to each person we met, patting the dogs that ran to greet us. Dogs seemed to be everywhere and enjoyed the same rights as the people who walked the street. There were a few cars, driven slowly around the people and around the dogs. And why not? No one was going anywhere he couldn't have walked to. We held hands as we scuffed through the dust, back to the pigeon. Zeballos would be our town, our headquarters for needed supplies and for service for the pigeon. We liked what we had seen.

Chapter 25

Leaving Zeballos to return to Seattle, we'd blown a jug, a vital part of our engine. At Kenmore we blew another jug. Bob Munroe, owner of Kenmore Air Harbor, suggested it could be a result of the strain put on our engine in our attempt to take the pigeon off Wabaska Lake. A new engine had to be installed. Its installation, and our determination to stop at the cove, delayed our work schedule in the North, but Wally was in high spirits.

"With a full load of gas out of Zeballos we can fly nonstop to Prince Rupert, which will cut down on our time."

True! But as we flew high over Sullivan Bay and Bella Bella, I looked down wistfully. "I feel like a traitor," I said.

"Yeah! I know." But he didn't stop.

Many changes had come with the eight years we'd been flying the coast. Herb Hetherington had just moved to Seattle and Al Baker was assuming the roll of sponsor. Ketchikan was changing, too. I missed those earlier, more leisurely days.

Betty King still paraded the streets in her bright orange coat, her dogs dancing around her.

Ageless, and salty as ever, she represented for me all that was best in Ketchikan. She gave it a certain stability. I met her on the street our first day in town.

"Mrs. Flynn," she greeted me, "damned if I didn't think you was never going to get here. Begging your pardon for the

language, Mrs. Flynn. And where is that husband of yours?"
She'd never quite forgiven him for sidetracking to Wabaska.
"I have business with him."

"He's around, Betty. You stop in at the clinic anytime.
He'll be glad to see you."

"And I'll be damned glad to see him. Begging your pardon!
I have a thing or two to say to that man. I told him to leave
me plenty of medicine last time he was here. Damned if he
didn't short me. Your pardon!" She paused, then admitted,
"Course, I didn't know the sons of . . . your pardon, in this
town were going to cast off so many."

"You tell him," I advised her.

"I am thanking you, Mrs. Flynn. You are good people, you
and your husband. I'll be in."

And she was in, several times, brightening our days. She
sassed and she scolded, and would always be something of an
enigma.

There were others who had stayed on in Ketchikan. The
madams we knew had mellowed with the years, their interest
now mainly in their pets. A new, more enterprising house had
flourished. We climbed the stairs together for our first call
there. Wally knocked at a door at the head of the stairs, and
a tiny window slid open, partially revealing a man's face. A bolt
was released, and the door swung open. An attractive woman
with flaming red hair was standing at the kitchen sink.

"My wife," the man said.

She nodded, and the man prodded us into the living room.
Two young women sat on the davenport, each holding a
Pomeranian. They could have been any two girls, except that
even though it was only mid-morning, they wore low-cut evening gowns.

"Honey! Sugar!" The man's introduction was brief.

They watched without comment as we trimmed the nails
and checked the ears and teeth of the Poms, but when we were
finished one of the girls opened a photograph album and held
it out to us.

"We always had German shepherds," she said. "Isn't he a

beauty? That's me between my brother and sister, and that's my mom."

Did I detect a sigh? Was this young woman perhaps missing her family? The other girl had also pulled out an album.

"Here's my family, Mom and Dad, and my younger brother, and there's Spunk, peskiest little cocker you ever laid eyes on."

These girls were lonely. They flipped the pages of their albums, showing us more pictures. But we had patients waiting at the clinic. The man showed us to the door and bolted it after us.

We worked long hours, until the day came to fly on to Sitka. With Wally engrossed in takeoff procedure, I compared our map to the misty terrain, seeking that channel that would keep us on course. Wally accepted my decision, but as we flew along, dodging the clouds, I became troubled. I studied my map and the terrain. They did not match. Wally growled at me, and I stiffened defensively.

"Where the hell are you taking us?"

"I don't know," I quavered.

"You don't know! What the hell kind of a navigator are you? You damn well better study that map and find out where we are."

Oh! I hated him. Yes, I had led us up the wrong channel, but how could I ever reconcile our position now? I yielded to a moment of terror. If our engine failed us, we'd never be found. I dared a glance at Wally. He showed no sign of weakening, just kept flying as though he knew where he was going. Maybe he did! I turned again to my map. Scud clouds that scurried in our path had begun to dissipate, and the terrain began to make sense.

"I know where we are!" I shouted triumphantly.

"About time!" But he made no effort to conceal a grin.

The louse! What he had known all along was clear to me now. Finding our way back through that maze of channels was impossible. Our only hope had been to fly west until the heavier swell indicated we were past the islands and then north until Baranof loomed ahead. He had deliberately taunted me, keeping me occupied in a search that made no allowances for panic. This man I had married was a most profound man. I reached out and squeezed his arm.

The feeling held, through busy days at Sitka, through the flight back to Ketchikan, with skies perfect and blue, the air smooth. Even the Tongass Narrows, usually turbulent, had succumbed to an uncommonly placid day. I watched idly as a seaplane took off some distance ahead of us. The pilot circled to a position behind us, then circled again, attaining a position off our left wing. Was this fellow playing games? I wondered uneasily. There was another abrupt turn.

"Wally! He's flying into us!"

Wally acted mechanically, flipping the pigeon onto her side and into a dive. Had the dazzling sun perhaps blinded that pilot? The engine of his plane passed over ours in such close proximity we could see the startled expression on his face.

"Couldn't we just once have a flight where nothing happens?" I asked shakily.

The cove, when we reached it, seemed a haven. I wished we'd never have to leave. At the same time, I looked forward to our return to Seattle. Maureen had written to us that she was engaged. She was home and had finished the semester. Dick, her fiancé, was in Korea, and they planned to be married when he returned.

When we arrived she greeted us somberly. "Gardenia's gone."

"Gone?" My mind refused to accepted the implication.

"Yes! We did everything, but we couldn't save her."

That pesky, obstinate, impossible creature! But I had loved her.

"She'd lived out her life, you know, and it was a good life." Wally paused and cleared his throat. "Yes, we'll miss her."

Maureen was unusually quiet those days as we sorted out supplies for our September clinic. She should have been excited about the resumption of fall classes, looking forward to seeing Jerry, her roommate. Could it be she missed Gardenia so much? Without her the rooms were too silent. Our departure day came, and still Maureen had given no indication of what was troubling her.

"Maureen," I said. "What is it?"

"Oh, Mother!" The words tumbled from her lips. "I worry so that something might happen, that you might never come back."

Our narrow escapes had been a never-failing source of conversation. Wally had refused to take them seriously, his sense of humor sending our listeners into gales of laughter—everyone except Maureen.

"Maureen, I didn't realize, but we can't let life frighten us. Every time you cross that street out front, there are cars whizzing by. Still you have to go across. It's the same with flying. We will come back. I promise you."

Her only answer was a tight little smile, and as we drove away I could see her standing there, watching. She was a young woman, but still my child. My heart ached for her. This trip north could not be too brief.

We stopped at the cove and at Zeballos for refueling, and this time, as we skipped over Sullivan Bay and Bella Bella, there were no qualms. Out of Bella Bella, however, we were met by strong head winds. Wally made rapid calculations. We'd be an hour overdue.

"Damn! I hate to be late. If we don't close our flight plan on schedule, somebody's going to worry."

"Let's just worry about getting there, shall we?" There was an edge to my voice that Wally didn't miss.

"What's eating you?"

"You know darn well. I hate the wind."

We maintained an altitude of three thousand feet until, on our way out of Grenville Channel, a high fog swirling in from the sea forced us down to a thousand feet. In the distance we could see Kaien Island.

As we flew up the channel that separates Kaien Island from the mainland, our engine coughed once, feebly—then silence! Seal Cove was clearly visible, less than three minutes away. At our reduced altitude, it was too far for a glide. The waters of the channel narrowed, cascading in a series of rapids, then widened to form Seal Cove. On a high tide these rapids were concealed, but now, from my side of the plane, they were very much in evidence.

"You'd better cut your glide," I observed dryly, "or you'll land us right in the rapids."

Our landing was uncomfortably close. The white waters lashed back, sucking at the pontoons. Wally was already out, paddle in hand, each stroke strong and determined.

"Keep on those foot pedals. Head her toward shore."

The current carried us across the channel, away from Prince Rupert. As our pontoons nudged the shore, Wally dropped into the water, holding us in.

He pointed up the bluff. "We'll have to climb halfway up to find a tree that will hold us." He tested each scrubby tree, finally choosing one he felt was sufficiently grounded. "There! And now let's see what happened."

Taking his measuring stick, he climbed up on the engine and over onto a wing, one, then the other. Both tanks were bone dry. Our gas gauge was unreliable. We should have had five hours' flying time. Our concern at the moment, however, was closing our flight plan. Prince Rupert wasn't on our frequency, and we were out of range of the Queen Charlottes. Wally decided to give Sandspit a try anyway.

I listened to his message: "Stinson N 14154 . . . Dr. Flynn, pilot . . . one passenger . . . down out of Prince Rupert. Need gas." He grinned, thumb and forefinger forming an O. "No injuries. We're okay until morning," and he repeated our position: "south of the rapids out of Seal Cove.

"Damned poor connection," he said to me, "but I think they got it."

It was six o'clock in the evening. We were complacent and warm in our cabin in spite of rain. But the rising tide was forcing us up a cliff that bristled with crags. Determined to keep our pontoons away from those menacing rocks, we plunged into the icy waters of the narrows.

Across the channel the lights of Prince Rupert gleamed

warmly, so near, yet beyond our reach. The bobbing head-lights of automobiles speeding along the opposite shore raised our spirits. Hoping an SOS might attract attention, we got out our high-beamed flashlight, sending one desperate signal after another, but the lights from the cars never wavered. We had flares and tried them, but they sputtered and died. As the hours passed those lights on the highway became fewer, and then there were none. Even the roar of the rapids was stilled, smothered too, in the depths of the sea.

It was a night of confusion, of floundering in the rising waters, stumbling over crags we couldn't see as the incoming tide forced us up the cliff. At tree level we encountered a new hazard. Gnarled branches threatened the wings. I stayed by the pontoons while Wally fought to keep the wings clear.

Six exhausting hours later, we were twenty feet up the cliff. The tide was changing and would force us no higher.

I found a log and lay down, and my eyes closed. I came to, bewildered and incoherent, facedown in the muck. Staggering back to the pigeon, I washed the mud from my face in the cold salty water. My hands were swollen, and my body ached. Clinging to the pontoon, I stared with morbid fascination at the black water swishing about my legs, harboring an irresistible urge to lie down and let myself be carried away, repelled yet attracted by the thought of release. Gradually, I became aware of the gentle lapping of the sea on the outgoing tide.

I turned to look for Wally. He said, "It won't be so bad going back down," and that was all the comfort he could offer.

I thought of Maureen and the promise I'd made. I thought of Mama and how, as a young woman driving a twenty-five-mile mail route out of Driscoll, North Dakota, she had fought to control a runaway team of horses frightened by lightning. I recalled our first day of school on the Montana prairies, when a sudden snowstorm had compelled her to walk the three miles to the country school to escort Berne and me home. The snow had blinded us, and we fell, to be helped to our feet by a mother who refused to give up. If they could see me now, sniffling away, how ashamed they would be!

We were hip deep in the icy water, and the chill September rain was persistent. The first pallid streaks of a new day relieved the blackness of night. The roar was like thunder, and in the wan gray light the swirling foam hissed and mocked us. Eight o'clock! The incoming tide had taken over again. How long until help would arrive?

Nine o'clock, and a plane flew overhead. At last! We waved; we shouted; but the plane gave no sign we'd been sighted. As we watched it disappear, the trauma of the long night swept over me, and I felt a sense of disbelief. Wally came to stand at my side and assured me: "Just a little while! Someone will come."

At ten o'clock, we spotted a tugboat advancing on the rapids, muted now by the rising tide. Could a boat navigate those treacherous waters? Breathlessly we watched as the tug hesitated and turned back, and our hearts sank. She approached again, and turned back. Why had they sent such a big boat, and why through the rapids? She approached a third time. She was in the rapids, caught up in the swirl, zigzagging, but steadily advancing. They'd made it. Their conquest brought a surge of energy I wouldn't have believed I could summon. I jumped up and down, shouting and waving, while the crew, with long pipe poles, tested for underwater crags, pulling in a few feet, testing again. With every foot our excitement mounted.

Wally was puzzled. "I can't understand why they didn't send a boat around the island to reach us from behind."

"I don't give a hang which way they came," I retorted. "I was never so glad to see a boat."

Then someone shouted, "Having trouble?"

We looked at each other. Certainly this was not the inquiry we had expected. But Wally was quick to answer. "We were expecting a boat to bring us some gas. Did you bring it?"

"No" was the puzzled reply. "Didn't hear about anyone needing gas, but if you're in trouble we'll do what we can to help."

If this boat wasn't sent to rescue us, one might still come, but neither of us felt inclined to wait.

"We've been here all night," Wally told them. "Could you get us some gas?"

Would they simply tell us they'd send someone else? We had waited so long. Sixteen wretched hours! If they went away . . . but the next words were beautiful.

"It would be much easier and faster to snug your plane alongside and take you right in to Seal Cove. If we snug her up tight, she should make it okay."

We didn't even stay on deck to see how our pigeon fared in the rapids. They took us below and gave us hot tea, and a half hour later we were in Seal Cove.

As we climbed from the tug, Viv Kellough raced down the ramp. Wet and dirty as we were, she put an arm around each of us. "You crazy darn kids! I knew it had to be you. Where were you?"

Wally scratched his head, nonplussed. "Just back of the rapids. Didn't Sandspit tell you?"

"They said someone, couldn't make out who, was forced down at South Rapids. We've spent the whole darn morning searching our maps for South Rapids. None of us ever heard of such a place."

Wally groaned. "Reception was bad, but I hoped I'd made it clear. Well, no matter, but didn't anyone see our SOS?"

"I did." One of the men on the ramp spoke up. "I just wondered what darn fool was playing around over there. Never dreamt anyone could be in trouble so close to town."

Viv drove us to the hotel. Later we began to puzzle over our empty tanks. In spite of a prolonged flight, there should have been gas to spare. We had seen the tanks spill over when we took on our gas load at Zeballos.

"You know," Wally said finally, "I don't believe she was full. It's like pouring water into a hot water bottle. If you pour too fast, the water bubbles over, but a vaccum has been created and there's still room at the top." It was the only logical answer.

A few days' rest and we were ready to go on. Not even a sniffle remained to remind us of our bout with the sea. The swelling had gone from our hands and feet, and even the irritating rash caused by long exposure to the salt water had disappeared. We worked long hard hours in Ketchikan and, on our return, in Prince Rupert. I was eager to be finished, to return to Seattle and see Maureen. I was impatient to keep the promise that had kept me going throughout our encounters.

Chapter 26

By March I sensed Wally was growing restless. "I'd like to get back to the cove," he said, "do some painting, get at some of those repairs. Ray Bailey wants to go along."

Ray Bailey, a neighbor, was an avid fisherman. He often stopped in just to talk fishing. I was immediately suspicious.

"So! You've been plotting behind my back. Are you guys going to work, or is this just a fishing trip?"

Wally's grin was a giveaway. "We'll probably fish a little."

"Okay. Just don't keep me waiting too long."

Though he promised, it was six weeks before I saw him again. His letters, however, recounted their activities, and I read them with amusement: "Dear Pinky, I like your color choice. Much better than brown! And wait until you see the windows we put in the doors. Lets the sun in for sure. We got a tramway built up the bluff and rigged up a cart with some iron wheels we found lying around. Father Lobsinger got us a winch in Zeballos. Sure helped with the mattress and the two upholstered rockers I ordered from Vancouver. Put them on the cart and zipped them right up the bluff. Oh, yes, we got a garden started. Things are popping up already. By the way, sure had us a dandy supper last night. Caught a red snapper."

My impatience to see for myself increased with each letter. My turn came at last. I raced up the bluff, to be stopped at the top by a glorious display, flowers blooming in unrivaled profusion, as though some giant hand had scattered seedlings at random. How fitting for a home in the forest.

Weeding the garden, hauling up wood, preparing a snapper for supper, we lost track of the days, even of the hour of the day. Evenings, we relaxed in our rockers, a roaring fire in the living-room heater providing cheerful insulation against a chilly night.

"Pinky," Wally said one night, "where's the catalogue?"

"You left it upstairs, I think. I'll get it." I ran up the stairs, but as I brushed by the chimney wall I felt heat. I touched it with my hand. "Wally! The chimney! It burns my hand."

He leaped from his chair and was out the door. I followed. Flames, a yellow glare against the black night, were leaping from our chimney, tossing sparks in a terrifying fireworks display.

"If those sparks land in the trees or on our dry shakes, we've had it. Thank God the rain barrels are full. I can get out on the porch roof from the upstairs window and climb up to the chimney. You keep the buckets of water coming."

I held my breath as his shoes scraped on the steep roof. He could fall, but there was no time to dwell on such thoughts. Upstairs and down! Buckets of water! We were able to control the fire, but it would not go out.

"Damn chimney must be full of pitch," Wally speculated. "Probably hasn't been cleaned in years. Should have thought of it when Ray was up. Well, it's burned clean now. We sure learn the hard way."

Up above the stars gleamed, tiny lamps in the night, and one by one blinked out, giving way to the gray of morning. The black smoke became a thin white wisp, and the sparks, faint and faltering, desisted at last. We sank into our chairs. The house was a shambles, reeking of smoke, tracked with water and cinders.

"My God!" Wally drew a trembling hand across his grimy forehead. "We can't even keep out of trouble sitting on the ground."

We made a few halfhearted attempts to swab up the worst, but the results hardly seemed worth the effort.

The next night not a sound disturbed the stillness, yet an uneasy feeling persisted. An aftermath of the preceding night? I had to be sure. Ignoring Wally's repeated warning never to move around at night without my flashlight, I shuffled down the hall to the stairs. It was a tricky stairway, no railing, narrow steps, and an L turn two-thirds of the way down. I stepped from the hall and off into space, somersaulting to the turn of the L, brought to a jarring halt by an unyielding log wall. I slid the remaining few steps, my head coming to rest on the living-room floor, my body sprawled on the steps. Wally was beside me.

"Don't scold me," I pleaded. "Please don't scold me."

He didn't scold. He didn't even ask how I could have been so foolish. He just slipped an arm under me and carried me up to bed.

I was not a pretty sight in the morning: a purple lump on my forehead, eyes swollen nearly shut, both knees twice their normal size.

"Can you walk?" Wally asked. I nodded. "Nothing's broken. I guess," he concluded.

I hated myself. Didn't we have enough problems without my adding one more? Wally was sick, I could tell. His face was pale, his hands trembled. I wanted to say something clever, something that would make our situation seem not quite so bleak, but I couldn't think of anything except that our lovely, freshly painted home had been reduced to a sooty mess. For the first time, we had given way to despair simultaneously. The day reflected our misery: gray skies and a steady drizzle. The house seemed to press in on me. By late afternoon I could stand it no longer. I made my way to the beach and stood there, unmindful of the rain, scanning the inlet. If only Father Lobsinger would come!

Then I heard a boat. It was Father Lobsinger!

He took one startled look at me. "By the heavens! Whatever happened to you?" There was no comment as I poured out my story. "You should be in hospital," he said. "I'll take you."

"I can't leave. Wally's sick."

"I'll stay the night then."

He bounded up the steps, but I remained on the beach, wondering. Had we been foolhardy, attempting to make a home where seeing another human was so altogether a matter of chance? The dampness and the late-afternoon chill penetrated my jacket. I shivered and turned to shuffle back to the house, my questions unresolved.

Certainly Father's presence had dispelled the gloom. The lamps were lit, and the old kitchen stove emitted a cheery warmth. Wally seemed to be more himself. I was to go to the hospital—both men were adamant.

X-rays in Seattle, later that week, disclosed a crack in one of the vertebrae, but I reacted vehemently to the doctor's suggestion of a brace. I could mend without it, he admitted, but I'd have to be grounded.

Not Wally. "I'm going back and get that place cleaned up," he said. "I'll give Allen Kasony a call. He said he'd like to help wire the house. We'll get a little generator, and when you come up, well, there'll be lights all over the house."

Three long weeks, but I was back. The house was so clean. Had we really had a fire? Then I looked up and saw a protective railing guarding the stairway. That night our castle glowed, lights streaming from every window. Yet, somehow, the flickering flame of our kerosene lamps seemed more in keeping with the old house. For us, the bright lights would be only an occasion.

Our work in the North was delayed until July to give my back more time to mend. At the cove again, Wally saw I was unusually quiet.

"Lonesome?" he asked.

"Sorta."

"Let's bring Maureen up for a week."

My eyes brightened, but then I remembered. "She's working."

"Well, it's time she had a vacation. If they won't let her off, she can quit. Never wanted her to work in the first place."

"Oh, but she wants to. All the kids work. But if she can get off . . ."

She did get time off, and the weather was ideal for our flight.

Her week went all too fast, but before she left she made an exciting disclosure. "You guys hurry home after your trip north in September, okay? Dick will be back from Korea in a couple of weeks. We plan to be married in October."

My inclination was to return to Seattle at once, but that wouldn't have been fair to our clients, and when I was back up north, working again with the animals, I was glad I hadn't given in to my whim. I was especially glad when we got a call from Lucy.

We had not been called to treat the birds, though she took us to visit them. It was Jim-Chin, her cat, she told us. He'd become such a problem.

I remembered when Jim-Chin was just a playful kitten, coal black with white chin whiskers, rather absurd. He looked as though he'd been dipped in a saucer of milk, hence the name. Now he was a grown cat, sleek and beautiful.

"But he won't stay home," Lucy protested. "Do you think he feels neglected or that maybe I don't love him? I do love him," she added quickly, "and I worry so about him. I'd feel terrible if anything happened to him like what happened to poor Casper. Such a gentle cat, he was, but he wandered off into the brush and a mountain beaver attacked him. At least we think it was a mountain beaver. He managed to crawl home, but he was all chewed up. Lee just had to do away with him.

"What do you think I should do, Dr. Flynn?"

"I think you should let us neuter him, Lucy. Otherwise he's going to keep roaming, and you'll keep worrying."

"I suppose you're right," she said thoughtfully. "Yes, of course you are right." She sighed. "He's so beautiful. I was hoping . . . well, if he mated with Agatha or Maybelle there would be such lovely kittens."

"Well, now," Wally suggested, "he just may have already."

She brightened visibly. "Yes. He could have. Oh, that would be nice. And of course, if he's going to be a father it's even more important that nothing happen to him."

With most of our clients the neutering of a male cat wouldn't have required a second thought, but with Lucy every decision was major.

And soon after, we were on our way to Seattle. So many things to do for the wedding. I seemed to be going in circles.

"Don't get yourself in such a stew," Wally admonished me. "It will all get done. It's going to be the loveliest wedding you ever saw."

Maureen and Dick were a handsome couple, but my eyes were on Wally that day, as he walked up the aisle with the girl he called daughter clinging demurely to his arm.

Chapter 27

"We've serious talking to do, Chicken." Wally drummed his fingers against the windowpane, staring out at the November rain. "We've been procrastinating, you know. Bob's really carrying the load here at the hospital. He'd like to buy it."

I frowned, biting my lip. "Do you want to sell?"

"No! Hell, I love this place. It . . . it all started here."

"Do we have to decide now?"

"No, Bob's not pushing us."

"Let's let it ride then, at least until we get used to the idea."

In our hearts we knew what that final decision would be. On the first day of February, 1959, we signed the papers that ended our reign at the hospital. It was not a happy day. In spite of a promise to stay on for a month, Wally begged for release.

"Let me go to the cove. I'll come back for you in March."

His letters came often. "Dear Pinky: Well, we've got a radiophone. Getting the aerial up was one hell of a job. Had to chop down a couple of trees that were in the way." He'd ramble on, but invariably the letters would end, "I miss you! I watch the sea gulls and the eagles. There's always two. A home is not a home with just one."

March came, and Wally was back. The movers had been in. Maureen had taken Minx. Vicki would go with us. "We're all set," I said with a grin, "except maybe Vicki. I don't think she's quite happy with all that's been going on around here."

He picked her up and snuggled her up against him. "We'd better put you in a carrier, I guess. You're probably not going to like that noisy old plane, either."

She didn't like it, and she liked the carrier even less. She pawed and scratched, and each pitiful whine ended in a sharp little yelp.

"She can't go on like that for three hours," I fussed. "She'll work herself into a heart attack."

"Do you think you can hold her? She'll be a handful."

"I'll hold her," I said as I released the catch. "Oops! Darn, you're fast, you rascal, but you're going to sit on my lap whether you like it or not."

Kneeling backward in my seat, I made a grab for the nape of her neck, but the pigeon lurched and I fell against Wally.

"Sorry, darling!"

"At a time like this!" Vicki whined softly, her brown eyes two pools of distrust. "Darn it! Any other time you'd beg to sit on my lap. And don't you laugh," I grumbled at Wally as I leaned over the back of the seat. "If you think I like standing on my head with you bumping all over the sky! Vicki, why can't you behave?" I made a dive for her, striking my head against a bulky object wrapped in plastic. "Ouch! What's that?"

"Just a little something I picked up at Kenmore."

I came up from behind my seat and eyed him suspiciously. "What is it?"

"I'll show you when we get home."

"I want to know now."

"Okay, it's an outboard, just a small one, five and a half horsepower."

"An outboard! We haven't even got a boat."

"Well, we could find one maybe."

With Vicki dancing at our feet when we reached the cove, we strolled up to the house. At the top of the steps a grouse emerged from the bushes. Yelping in delight, Vickie was after her. The grouse easily evaded her tormentor, coming to rest in the branches of a filbert tree.

"Vicki!" Wally's voice was stern. "Leave Minniebelle alone.

You learn to get along, or you'll wind up in a peck of trouble. Minniebelle's special," he explained to me. "Been hanging around this whole month I've been alone."

Minniebelle *was* special, I found. She'd dart across our path or light in a filbert tree, nodding approval as we dug and planted our garden. When the tiny plants poked through the sod and I knelt on the ground, weeding, she'd perch in the plum tree, tossing down at me an occasional hard pellet of a plum. If we stayed indoors too long, we could expect her to stomp the full length of our kitchen roof.

"We're going to have to tear this damned porch down," Wally swore one day as he came out with a tiny hummingbird clutched in his hand. "They wander in there, then can't find their way out. This little guy would have beat himself to death against the window if I hadn't caught him."

Released, he flew upward, returning with lightning speed on a direct head-on course, swerving just in time to zip past the top of Wally's ear, all the while emitting that strange wild call.

The day I caught Wally slipping cardboard under a length of stovepipe in the storage room, I was not so sympathetic. I watched in astonished disbelief as he carried the entire ensemble outside and lifted the pipe, allowing one thoroughly frightened little mouse to scurry to freedom.

"Honestly! That little beggar will be right back inside."

"I know," Wally admitted sheepishly, "but with those little eyes pleading up at me I couldn't do away with him."

That pipe seemed to attract mice. Some time later I found three pair of eyes pleading with me. "Don't you dare look," I threatened Wally. "I'll dispose of these myself."

There was no lack of activity, but there was special excitement the day Father Lobsinger came in. He was waving a package.

"Hey!" he yelled. "Appears you ordered some rosebushes."

"Right!" Wally yelled back. "We're going to grow the best in the country. Come on up. Must be about lunchtime."

Father anchored his cruiser and came ashore in the eight-foot skiff he carried aboard the larger boat.

"That's a dandy little skiff," Wally observed. "If you run across one like it for sale, let me know. I brought an outboard up from Seattle, but it doesn't do us much good without a boat."

"Not much," Father Lobsinger agreed. "How would you like this one? It's plain too heavy to be dragging on and off my cruiser. I'll drop this one off for you as soon as I can get a new one."

So before long we had a boat, but Father's return visit had a dual purpose. Bill Robertson, a fisherman who lived about a half mile on past Nuchatlitz, had an Airedale he wanted Wally to have a look at. "I'll run you over," Father said.

They let me off at Nuchatlitz. They weren't gone long, and I didn't think to ask about the dog. I was thinking of matters Rose Michael and I had discussed. The children had terrible sores. Wally agreed we could probably do something about it, but first he had to check with Dr. McLean at the small mission hospital at Esperanza.

"I don't want to overstep any bounds," he said.

A few days later I had cause to remember the dog. We were on the beach. Wally seemed to be studying the chop of the waves with more than usual interest. When he turned to me, his voice was casual. "Guess I'll run over to the Robertsons' and have another look at that female." It was nothing too serious, he explained. She'd had pups some while back, a large litter. Nursing so many had taken a lot out of her.

"Great. I'd like to meet the Robertsons."

"Not this time, Chicken," he said. "I'm taking the skiff."

"It's too rough out there for a little boat," I protested. "What's wrong with flying?"

"Bill doesn't have a tie-down for a plane yet."

"Sounds fishy to me, after all the places we've landed! But if you're bound to go in the boat, I'll go along."

"Uh-uh! One in the boat in this sea is okay, but not two. Now don't worry. I'll look at the dog and come straight home."

It would be two hours before I could hope for Wally's return, but I could not leave the beach. At last, the sound of an engine, and I saw a speck on the water coming closer, closer.

"I did it!" Wally crowed as he pulled into shore, and I realized the skiff and the sea had been a challenge he couldn't resist. He promised me we'd get a bigger boat.

That trip to Bill's was the start of a new venture. Bill had spread the word. He stopped by the following week. "They want you in Zeballos, Doc," he called from his troller.

Ah, that was great. Zeballos, our town, now even more our town. We had a few spays and castrations, but not as many as we had come to expect. Zeballos was cut off from the outside world, their only contact by seaplane or freighter. With un- limited space, the few families living there were indifferent to the number of dogs that roamed their street. It was exciting to have an animal doctor at their command. Certain conditions we were called upon to treat were so incidental we felt sure our good neighbors had extended themselves to find something wrong with their pets. There were enough serious cases, how- ever, to make us feel good about our Zeballos practice.

We hadn't forgotten Rose and the dreadful sores on the children's arms and legs, and we made a trip to the mission hospital at Esperanza to talk with Dr. McLean. Esperanza was about thirteen miles from the cove, on a channel branch- ing off Esperanza Inlet. Esperanza had no store and could not rightly be called a village. There was a two-story frame hos- pital, actually just a very large house, and a number of smaller houses, homes of those who worked at the hospital.

Dr. McLean was more than willing to have us do what we could for the Indian people at Nuchatlitz. The area was large, and he couldn't get around to the villages as often as he would have liked. He was the mysterious owner of that lovely little cottage across the cove. He gave no indication he wanted to sell, but I hoped he just might be so inclined. I could dream.

In the meantime, Nuchatlitz became, in a sense, our re- sponsibility as our Indian neighbors came with their prob- lems. It was a reciprocal relationship fostering mutual respect. We gave Chief Felix the B vitamins he needed.

"I'll sharpen your saws," he offered in return.

Frank Savey had no special request, but he came anyway. We were having lunch and weren't aware we had company until we saw him looking through the window in the kitchen door. I invited him to join us and he came in, but he merely toyed with his food. This puzzled me.

Finally he spoke. "My wife would like this."

"Your wife? Where is she?"

"She waits in the boat."

Sophie, like many of the older Indian women, spoke no English except for "Yes" and "No," but there was a matter of protocol. An invitation must be extended before she would step from that boat, an invitation she was eager to accept. She chatted happily while she ate, words that made no sense to me. Her round face was wrinkled in smiles, and her warm brown eyes sparkled.

When they were ready to leave, we walked with them down to the beach. Sophie was thin and wiry. In spite of her age, which I judged to be around seventy, she ran down the steps. Frank took them more slowly. He was taller than Wally and somewhat heavy. Sophie held their old dugout canoe steady while he climbed in and sat in the stern. She took her place beside the inboard and with a rope she pulled and pulled. Frank watched her placidly.

One day Bill came again. We watched, amazed, as he dropped four ungainly Airedale pups into his skiff and rowed them to shore.

"Hi, Doc, Mrs. They're females. I want them spayed."

I liked him.

Others followed Bill's example, bringing their pets to us. A man from Tahsis came in a speedboat, bringing a Labrador with a severe upset stomach. Tahsis was a mill town with a population of about fifteen hundred. They wanted us in Tahsis, he told us. Then there was a call to Tofino, seventy miles south of us. In between our calls patients continued to arrive at the cove, by troller, even by chartered seaplane.

"Who would have believed it!" Wally marveled. "We aren't retired. We've not even semiretired."

One night while we slept, thousands of sea gulls converged on our islands, coming to rest on the gnarled branches of wind-blown evergreens.

"Whatever brought them?"

"Beats me!" Wally replied. "Maybe if we go down to the beach we'll find the answer."

I ran ahead, then stopped, stunned. Our limpid green waters, which revealed rocks on the bottom and sea grasses responding to the movement of tides, had taken on a new hue and consistency, a milky green opaqueness. The beach was equally astonishing, glistening frostily in the morning sun, but the mysterious substance that coated every rock and pebble was not frost. Wally knelt to examine the slippery particles.

"They're fish eggs. The herring must have spawned. That accounts for the sea gulls. They've come for the feast."

And they stayed, piercing the air with their screams. We watched them, treading gingerly over the rocks. Would those noisy scavengers never get their fill? Finally, one of the seals lurking amid the underwater crags seized the leg of a sea gull, which disappeared for all time.

One afternoon, having returned to the house for a hasty lunch, we became aware of more sonorous sounds mingled with the screams. There were bellows of rage, or was it fear?

"Come on," Wally yelled, grabbing up a sandwich. "We're missing something."

The seals had taken off, replaced by sea lions, which, though similar in appearance, were more ponderous. They had singled out one unwary member from a pack of killer whales, or maybe he was old and sick and had been deserted. In any event, they had him encircled between our outer beach and a small island three hundred yards away. The past several days we had observed these whales leaping in play in the lee of an island near the Owasitsa River, their pointed tail fins cutting through the water with alarming speed.

Now the battle was on. The slap of the black body as it alternately leaped and dove, churning the water, and the roars of the attackers combined to drown out the screams of the gulls. Though the whale was hopelessly outnumbered, for we counted eight sea lion heads surfaced simultaneously, he was a powerful adversary, and our sympathies were with him. We sat spellbound, unaware of our own shouts of encouragement. It took a full two hours to defeat him. He made one last lunge, then plunged into the sea and did not reappear. Gone, too, were the sea lions, not even a ripple to suggest their presence. The sudden silence was startling. We sat staring at the water, now so calm. Had we really witnessed a battle?

"My God!" Wally brushed his hand across his forehead as if to break a spell. "What a magnificent creature!"

The battle was the climax in our episode of the herring. The seals, the sea lions, the killer whale all disappeared, seeking deeper water and other prey. Even our obstreperous gulls took off, except those few too lethargic to move on. The changing tides had cleansed our rocks of the remaining eggs; the water in our cove returned to its normal pellucid complexion. The show was over.

Chapter 28

I poked tentatively at an inoffensive little weed, but the sun was so hot. I stretched out on my stomach, laid my head in the crook of my arm. I was almost asleep when a movement in the tall grass alerted me and I found myself staring into the beady eyes of a garter snake. The head disappeared in the grass, then reappeared, the little forked tongue darting in and out.

But I was so sleepy. "Beat it, Jimmy! I was here first." With that ultimatum, I shut my eyes. Moments later I felt it slither along my bare arm.

"You win!" I jumped to my feet and went down to the beach, where snakes were not so apt to be slithering about. Wally found me there some while later.

"Hey! I thought you were weeding."

"I was . . . sort of, but those darn snakes! I don't like them sneaking up on me when I'm sleeping."

"Sleeping, eh?" Wally's eyes twinkled. In all probability, he had been napping too. "By the way, do you know what day's coming up?"

"I don't even know what today is."

He tipped his head back and let the laughter roll out. "You're bushed, no two ways about it."

"Bushed?"

"Yep! That's what they call it here when you don't know what day it is and don't care. Then it's time to get back to civilization. How would you like to spend Mother's Day with Maureen?"

Maureen was seven months pregnant, expecting, she insisted, a son, and Wally agreed that if Maureen said it was going to be a boy, it would be a boy. I preferred a wait-and-see attitude.

On our way back we stopped in Vancouver to pick out the larger boat Wally had promised me. We settled on a fourteen-foot clinker-built rowboat with a small inboard. It would be delivered at Zeballos via the *Tahsis Prince*, a freighter that made weekly trips up the west coast of the island.

Even more exciting, we contacted the widow of Stanley Newton. Ever since that first day we'd poked around in the ruins of the old post office, Wally had been determined to learn more about the people who had settled there first. Gertrude's memories were as vivid as if she'd never been away from the cove. She told us that the Newton family—father, two sons, Stanley and Gordon, and a daughter, Anna—had come from England to settle in Saskatchewan after the death of the mother. Unable to adjust to the prairie climate, they moved to the Pacific coast. Stanley eventually found work in a store at Hot Springs Cove, about fifty miles south of our cove. In a small rowboat Stanley set out to explore Nootka Island, which had been opened to homesteading, and came upon the cove. In 1914 the family joined him and the old log house, now ours, was built.

She told how other homesteaders had come and gone, unable to survive the harsh wilderness country. The Newtons had persevered, sustained by the store and the post office. Their supplies had come up the coast on the old steamship *Maquinna* on its irregular runs, often three weeks apart. It anchored out in the inlet, and the men rowed out in a dory to meet it. The Indians and a few trappers and fishermen had been their customers.

At that time there was no Zeballos or Tahsis or Esperanza. Then the discovery of gold had brought people to the Zeballos area, and for a time Zeballos had flourished. Logging had

been responsible for the establishment of Tahsis. Esperanza
had come later. Dr. McLean had been searching for an out-
post area and had found it at Esperanza.

In 1922 the cottage was built for Gordon Newton's bride.
I told Gertrude how much I loved that little cottage, and
that I'd wanted it from the first moment I'd seen it.

"Why don't you buy it?" she asked. "Miss Langdale wanted
our property, but Dr. McLean just more or less took the
cottage off Ada's hands when Gordon died. I'm sure the doctor
never intends to live there. You could double what he paid
and it would still be a bargain. Land up there hasn't much
value yet. People don't want to be that isolated." She paused
a moment, then added, "I've been hoping there might be a tie
of sorts between us. My niece's sister-in-law in California has
a sister living somewhere up the coast. I thought it might be
you folks, but the husband is a veterinarian, and you're a
dentist, aren't you?" she asked, turning to Wally.

"No," he replied. "I'm a veterinarian."

"You are? Then maybe you are the people. Ellen, my niece,
speaks so often of Bernadene."

"That's my sister!" I squealed.

"And if Jack hadn't prodded us, we probably never would
have bought the place," Wally added.

On the way home I reflected on our visit with Gertrude. It
seemed only right that the cove should be ours, and that included the cottage.

We stopped in Zeballos before going on out to the cove.
No one was at the ramp, so we headed up the street. Not a
soul on the street, either, and every door was shut. It was as
if the town had been evacuated. Then we spotted a man
coming around the corner of a house.

"Hello!" Wally bellowed. "Where is everybody?"

"Up the valley at the ball game," he replied. "Had to come
back for some drinks. Celebrating the Queen's birthday."

He didn't tarry. Evidently "up the valley" there was a great
thirst. We didn't tarry, either, stopping only long enough to
pick up the mail from our box. One letter puzzled me. The

precise handwriting was surely Miss Langdale's, but the name didn't fit, and the return address was a convent in England. There was no time to read it then, but I ripped it open as soon as we were home.

It *was* from Miss Langdale, and she *was* in a convent. I read with increasing amazement. Not only had Miss Langdale entered a convent, she had joined a contemplative order where strict silence was sternly maintained. I thought of her that day we'd first come to the cove—a nonstop talker, a chattering wren. Her new vocation seemed too unlike her nature, and I could hardly accept it. As I read on, I realized she, too, found it difficult to accept. No matter how hard she tried, she ended up speaking. I sensed her discouragement, and a gnawing loneliness.

Another letter, about a week later, explained in detail. Mrs. Ball had family and friends. She'd had no problem adjusting to city living. But Miss Langdale, a spinster, had no family, and her only friends were the Indian people she'd lived and worked with for so many years. She felt lost and alone in Vancouver with people she couldn't relate to. In a convent, she had thought, she would be safe from the perplexities of the world. There would be no distressing decisions to make. She had acted without taking into consideration her gregarious inclinations. Yet she stayed on, praying for a miracle that would change her into the person she had thought she could be. I answered her letters. She needed a friend, maybe only a sounding board, but I filled the need.

Hardly a day passed that I didn't wander over to the cottage, to peek in the windows, to admire the mahogany paneling in the living room and kitchen and the papered walls in the bedroom. I anticipated the autumn sweetness of tiny green grapes in the greenhouse. I climbed the flower-lined rock steps behind the house, which led to the top of the bluff, and gazed out over the inlet, but always my gaze returned to rest on the cottage.

One day I came back from the cottage determined to ask Wally why we didn't go to Dr. McLean at once to see if he would sell. I found Wally behind the house, with a tub of water, giving Vicki a bath. He'd pour water over her with a pan. She'd shake, splattering him all over. It was a ridiculous scene, but they were having great fun, neither of them minding the wetness. I laughed, watching them; then suddenly a startling realization took hold of me. I had wondered sometimes if Wally was completely happy here, if he ever regretted having sold the hospital. I saw now, by the light in his eyes, that his happiness was complete, but I wanted to hear the words.

"You like it here," I said, a statement rather than a question.

"Right, Chicken! It'll be a good long time before anyone fences us in here."

I knew what he was referring to. In Seattle, commercial establishments had sprung up on either side of us and across the street. He had felt crowded. Here at the cove we breathed freedom. I forgot about the cottage temporarily.

Chapter 29

The afternoon sun was hot. Sweat beaded on Wally's fore-head and trickled down his face, but he did not pause in his work. A float for the pigeon had to be finished before the tide would sweep in, undermining our efforts. The building of the float had been given top priority. Salt water rusts aluminum pontoons. The pigeon must be brought up onto the float, where we could wash the salt off with fresh water from our streams. There was yet another reason for urgency. We were scheduled to leave shortly for our clinics in the North. That would take us into July, and in the latter part of July Mau-reen's baby was due. We wanted to be in Seattle by then.

We'd salvaged boards and planks from the sea and had chosen the southeast corner of the cove, where the wind seldom hit. We'd build at the half-tide mark, which would give us more leeway for coming and going. The float, anchored at the four corners with six-foot lengths of nylon rope secured to anchors, or deadmen, buried deep in the gravel, would allow our float to accommodate to the rise and fall of the tides.

Nailing the float together hadn't been too difficult, but holes had to be dug and the deadmen buried before the sea took over. One deadman was an old iron wheel, another a ship's anchor. They took sizable holes. The sands shifted, rocks spilled into the holes, and the sea was relentless in its forward march.

"We won!" Wally exulted at last, throwing down his shovel. He pulled out a handkerchief and mopped his forehead. "Whew! Damn glad to get that job under my belt before we head up to Alaska."

Our Alaska itinerary this time would include Wrangell. We'd had a letter concerning a Labrador with an ear condition that could require surgery. There was no hotel in Wrangell, the letter advised, but there was a boardinghouse up from the dock.

"We'll hit Wrangell first," Wally decided. "It's most urgent."

The long trek up the inside passage had become standard procedure. We left the pigeon at the dock in Wrangell and sauntered along a wooden walk until we came to a large house surrounded by a white picket fence. A splash of flowers brightened its weathered exterior and a sign in the window proclaimed, BOARD AND ROOM. A pleasant-faced woman answered our ring.

"Well! You must be the doctor," she said. "You fit the description. We've been expecting you." As she talked she led us up a flight of steps and showed us to a room. "Just call me Billie," she said, then added, "I'll give Jim a call. He's mighty concerned about that Lab."

Smiling, she backed from the room, and we heard her footsteps on the stairs. We were not alone long. The fragrance of freshly brewed coffee alerted us even before the sound of her voice carried up the stairs.

"Coffee's ready! And Jim's here."

"Sure glad you're here, folks," Jim exclaimed as we sat down. He hesitated, then blurted out, "We've hit a snag, though, Doc. There isn't a vacant building in town, except one, if you didn't object." He hesitated again. "It's the jail. They said you'd be welcome."

"Doc's not going to jail." Our landlady's voice flared in indignation. "We'll have the clinic right here. I'll shove the furniture around a bit and roll the rug back. No trouble at all."

"Thank you, no!" Wally told her. "Your boarders would object to the ether, not to mention other assorted smells."

"Anyone doesn't like the smell can just leave." Her resolution was unshakable. "It's going to be here, and my two little Pekingese will be your first patients."

Jim was grinning. "It's settled. And don't worry about the boarders. Billie's got a monopoly."

If the boarders didn't object, Billie's Pekingese did, especially the female, her double set of tiny white teeth flashing as she snarled in protest.

"The baby teeth never did come out," Billie explained. "Doesn't seem to bother except when she's eating."

But both sets were avid for a nip at my hand. Wally gave the injection, and while she slept we relieved her of that unnecessary adjunct to her defiance mechanism. The defiance, however, remained unchanged. When she awoke, still groggy, the lip curled as if to say, "I'll get you for this."

I picked her up, taking care to elude those remaining teeth. "Hey, you little rascal, we're your friends." She was not immediately convinced, but before we left Wrangell she had taken over not only us but our room, darting in whenever the door was ajar.

Jim's Labrador was her exact opposite, friendly and cooperative from start to finish, realizing, with some sixth sense, that we meant to help him.

Billie's boardinghouse soon did smell like a hospital, but if anyone complained to her it did them no good. She accepted the disruption of boardinghouse routine with smiling aplomb.

The summer rains didn't materialize those weeks we were in Alaska. People tired quickly, and became irritated too easily. It was hot when we returned to the cove, and one by one our streams were reduced to a trickle.

"Might be some water in that old well back of the house," Wally suggested.

It was shallow, maybe five feet deep. The water had looked murky when we'd peeked in, in the spring, but now we couldn't be choosy. Off came the lid. It was bone dry, and a huge grandfather frog blinked in protest against the sudden sunlight. He hopped twice, croaking indignation at this invasion of his privacy.

"Are you all right down there?" Wally's call was answered by another croak.

There seemed no way he could have entered or could leave, but he showed no signs of starvation or dehydration. At least it was cool down there. We replaced the lid and left him to his meditations.

I suspected there'd still be a trickle in the far stream. I trudged on to the third. There'd been a fair trickle here only yesterday. Now, not a drop. Looking from the dry bedrock to my empty bucket, I was suddenly overwhelmed by the hopelessness of it all. I sat on the rocks, my chin resting on my knees, my hands clasped about my ankles, and I cried. However could we stay here with no water? Wally found me there, hunched on the rocks, crying.

"That's no way to act," he reproached me. "We'll find water."

"There isn't any," I wailed, and my tears flowed anew.

Wiping my eyes, I got to my feet and followed him, back to the second stream, back through the crackling brush, and up the exposed rocks to the very top of the waterfall. There we found a patch of moss. It was wet and spongy when we pressed it with our hands.

"There's water here," Wally announced triumphantly. "Must come from some underground pocket. Wait here."

He went down the waterfall at breakneck speed and was soon back with a pair of tin snips and a piece of aluminum sheeting. He cut it to form a spout and anchored it in the moss. I balanced my bucket on the rocks under the spout. Drip! Drip! With measured precision the precious fluid tinkled into our bucket. The minutes ticked by, twenty, thirty, thirty-five. Our bucket was full.

In the days that followed it seemed our demand must surely exceed our supply, but the drip remained constant. We had been forty days without rain.

Then it came. It came in torrents. It filled our streams, sending them thundering over the rocks, overflowing in rivulets all over the beach in their mad rush to the sea.

Wally realized we must find a way to hold back that rush of water, but for me the crisis was over. My mind was occupied with another matter. We knew the arrival of Maureen's baby was imminent.

"Don't you think it's time we were getting down to Seattle?" I demanded one lazy afternoon.

"What's the rush? The baby isn't due yet."

"It could come early, you know."

"Oh, honestly!" He was as excited about that baby as I, but at times he could be utterly exasperating.

Maureen did wait for us. Baby Gregory put in an appearance on August 2, late in the afternoon. A boy! Maureen and Wally had been right. I was delighted. We loved every demand this small baby could make. Fortunately for the young parents, our September schedule relieved them of the hampering ministrations of two overanxious grandparents.

Chapter 30

The log was a prize, at least sixty feet long and riding high in the water, almost certainly dry inside. Wally eased the skiff alongside and I pounded in a nail, bending the head over my rope and into the log. We needed that log for our winter's supply of wood. During the summer drift logs had been scarce, but now the higher tides lifted them from hidden beaches and fall winds eased them into the inlet.

Wally started the inboard, but as our boat inched forward our log rolled and swung, pulling me from my seat. I knelt, bracing my knees against the backboard, my arms straining in their sockets.

"Let out the slack," Wally sang out, his back to me.

"What slack?" I yelled back.

A quick look convinced him the only slack was my body. "You planning on a swim off the end of that log? Let her go."

"No! She's ours."

"Don't be silly. Both the wind and the tide are against us. I should have my head examined for trying it in the first place."

"I don't care. I'm not letting her go."

"You are a mule! Well, let's see if we can nudge her in."

It pulled us sideways and in circles, but we nudged and we prodded, teasing it into the cove. It was ours, ours to cut and slab and winch up the bluff to our woodshed.

Other chores were not so wearing. We picked berries, and as we worked our glances strayed to the cottage. The longing to own it had not diminished, but Dr. McLean had not been out, nor had we had occasion to go to Esperanza. No one would be looking for property up here anyway, certainly not at this time of year. Except Miss Langdale!

Her last letter had given us a jolt. Too much contemplating and too much praying had brought on a new distress. The world most surely was coming to an end. The only place where one might possibly escape the holocaust was the cove. Would we sell her back five acres so when it happened she would have a place to flee to? How she could flee from England in time to escape a sudden holocaust I couldn't imagine, but I didn't mention that when I wrote. I did tell her we didn't feel the world was coming to an end just yet and that we really didn't want to sell five acres, but that she was welcome to come and stay with us if she was worried.

The next letter was not from Miss Langdale but from the Mother Superior of the convent. Miss Langdale had been advised to leave their order, she stated. She was too old to adjust to their rigorous way of life, and she had gone to a convent that was less restrictive. We were not told where, nor did we hear from Miss Langdale again. We hoped that in a more lenient order she had at last found peace and security.

One day when I was preparing berries for jelly, Wally called from the beach. "Come on down. We have a visitor."

Setting the berries aside, I ran down. There was no boat. I saw no one. "Whatever are you talking about?" I demanded.

"There!" Wally pointed. "See him? How are you, Oscar?"

I did see him. He craned his neck, looking us over. Oscar was a remarkably friendly seal. He reveled in surfacing unexpectedly, managing with uncanny instinct to face us. He came again and again, his visits the highlight of the day. We anticipated his coming, worried if he was late. Then one day he brought a lady friend, and she also came to stay.

They were not our only companions. Many sea gulls came and went, but Reuben and Rachel remained constant. They were noisy, those two, screaming for attention. They followed us when we went fishing, demanding a share. It was wet and cold out there on the water, and they were a nuisance.

In November winds ripped through our trees with a roar as of jets. Though we feared for our pigeon on her homemade float, she rode out each storm with solid dignity. Then a new worry. Tossed by high seas and driven by the winds, massive logs assailed our cove. Pike poles in hand, we defended the pigeon, thankful for the outgoing tide, which gave us a respite. Even in the night we were on duty, flashlight in one hand, pike pole in the other.

"We're going to have to take her out," Wally declared.

We didn't act soon enough. On December 19 an entire tree marched in, branches protruding in all directions. We stuffed a few things into a bag, grabbed Vicki, and ran to free the pigeon. The tree was at our tail as we taxied from the cove. In the inlet we swung out of its path and caught our breath, though Wally was still fretting. There was too much ice on our wings.

"Where are we going anyway?" I demanded.

"To Seattle, after we drop Vicki off at Bill's. There's no safe place up here for a pigeon."

We'd be with Maureen for Christmas. I liked the idea. But the pigeon gave us a bad ride, resisting the controls, pulling to the side. We held over the water as much as possible, relieved when we spotted Pat Bay, where we decided to stay the night.

"I'm taking no chances on floating around out here in the dark," Wally declared. "Want to give Bob Munroe a call at Kenmore, too. Maybe he can advise us."

Bob did. "Could be water in the fuel line. Hard to say. Anyway, keep in radio contact when you fly down tomorrow. If you're forced down, we'll know where to look for you."

Our pigeon didn't let us down, but we were happy to turn her over to Bob. Whatever her problems, he would have ample time to correct them before we picked her up again in the spring. For the present, concerns were put aside. Christmas had never been more exciting. There was a gaiety far exceeding the occasion. Gifts flowed out from under the tree and around the room. In the short time allotted him Wally had gone on an all-out spending spree, or else he'd waylaid Santa.

When we left a few days after Christmas, I was glad. It had been a happy time, yet a strange feeling persisted. Could it be just that I wanted to go home?

What had been a three-hour flight became now a three-day journey. We took the train to Vancouver, staying the night with Al and Lavone, reminiscing over Clowholm days. And we sent a radiogram to Bill: MEET US IN ZEBALLOS JANUARY FIRST. The early-morning ferry, the following day, took us to Nanaimo on Vancouver Island.

"Low and slow!" Wally laughed. "It's taking us two hours to navigate a stretch of water we usually cross in twenty minutes."

At Nanaimo we transferred to a bus for Campbell River, a town located about two-thirds of the way up the east coast of the island. Then we transferred again, this time to a rattletrap bus which would take us through the mountainous interior of the island to the Gold River logging camp at the head of Muchalot Inlet on the west coast.

The bus wasn't crowded. There were eleven young men, dressed in boots and rough, warm clothing. The bus driver walked down the aisle with a sheet of paper, which each man signed with a casual indifference. Then he came to us. We read it together. Neither the logging company nor the bus company could be held responsible for any accident or unforeseen happening. Wally shrugged. He signed. So did I.

"By the way," Wally asked, "how far is it to Gold River?"

"Well—" The driver hesitated, seeming to consider. "Some say sixty miles, thereabouts, but by the time I've driven in and out of every damn rut I reckon you'll swear it's at least twice that."

We drove along a paved road for maybe twenty miles. Had the driver been kidding? The men lolled in their seats, smoking, joking.

"Thought you weren't coming back," one said to another.

"Hell!" was the reply. "Blew the whole damn lot of it. Got to make me another stake."

"Yeah! Same here. You going back to the same camp?"

"Why not? The boss'll be beefin' for me. 'Bout half of us walked out our last pay."

My attention was diverted by a steel gate barring our way. A watchman appeared, talked to our driver, then went to open the gate.

"Okay, you guys," the driver shouted. "Stamp out them cigarettes. You know damn well there's no smoking in company territory. Anyone lights up other side of this gate gets it rammed down his throat."

Cigarettes were tossed to the floor, ground to bits under heavy heels. The gate clanged after us. A narrow dirt road, blasted from rock walls, dropped precipitously on its outer edge. I stared down, hundreds of feet, and sucked in my breath. We lurched over rocks and in and out of ruts, skidded in the mud around hairpin turns, the front wheels pulling to the rock wall, the back wheels to the drop. Fine streams of water plunged down the walls and across the road, sluicing out more dirt and rocks. I was jostled from one hip to the other. Feet braced, I dug into my seat, pushing with outstretched arms against the seat in front.

"How's it going?" Wally asked. I could only shake my head.

I glanced at our traveling companions. Their faces were unreadable. How could any of them sleep? Yet some did, their heads bouncing against their chests with the regularity of a yo-yo. One fellow, wide awake, pointed to a car over the bank by a narrow bridge.

"Turned off to let the bridge go by," he observed, with no show of concern.

We came upon a car sideways across the road. Our driver was irate. "Where the hell does he think he's going?" He jumped from the bus to confront the other driver. "How many coupons did you send in to get your license? Which way you going anyway?"

And finally, Gold River campsite. It was six o'clock, dark

and cold and still raining. Slim Beale was waiting at the dock in his small water taxi. We piled on, arranging ourselves on benches on either side of the cabin, squeezed in so tightly even the crossing and uncrossing of one's legs was restricted. The men pulled cigarettes from shirt pockets and lit up, puffing dispassionately, and smoke hung in the air like a veil. My eyes stung, and the odor of too many bodies in too close confinement offended my empty stomach. It rumbled disconsolately.

"Thought carrying extra provisions was only for the pigeon." Wally spoke close to my ear. "Never dreamt there wouldn't be one stop for food this whole damned route."

The rain beat on the windows, harmonizing in a peculiar way with the *slap, slap, slap* of our boat as it bucked each oncoming wave. Now and again a dim light appeared in the night. As our taxi pulled in to an unseen dock, one of the passengers would struggle from his seat and, hunching his shoulders against the rain, disappear into the night, reporting for work at some isolated logging camp. It was ten o'clock when we reached Tahsis.

"How about a coffee break, folks?" Slim suggested. "There's a café up the road where you can get a hamburger, if you don't mind getting out in the rain. We'll be another hour getting to Zeballos."

We stood up and stretched, then stepped out into the night, our lungs responding to the sweetness of rain-washed air. In the café odors of another kind greeted us, the fragrance of coffee and the smell of fried onions.

As we were finishing our hamburgers, a sudden wind whipped up the night. I heard it screech around the corner of the café. Bent double against the wind and a deluge of rain, we raced for the boat. We were the only passengers continuing on to Zeballos. It was a wild, rough ride. Our boat sprang from the water as it rose to the crest of each choppy wave, returning with a shuddering crash that kept us out of our seats. A silvery spray shot high into the night, feathering our windows. We tried looking out, but could see nothing.

"Mite rough," Slim observed dryly.

Midnight, and the dim dock lights of Zeballos punctured the night. We could make out the black hulls of trollers anchored alongside the dock, bobbing like corks in the angry sea.

"Hell!" Slim swore. "Wouldn't you know there wouldn't be one damn hole where we could snake in? Hold us in, Doc. I'll tie alongside this troller."

Wally took the wheel, and Slim, rope in hand, sprang to the deck of the troller, snugging our taxi fore and aft.

"Hand over your bags, Doc," he shouted above the wind. "Now grab that flashlight off the ledge and take it easy as you come over the side. These boats damn well aren't going to sit still for you. Here," he said to me, "take my hand, and for God's sake watch where you're going. Don't go tripping over any lines."

I'm not sure how I made it onto the deck. The boats pitched and strained against the ropes.

"Nice night for a stroll, eh? I'll give you a hand with your bags to the hotel."

Wally objected. "We can make it."

"Hell, Doc, it's a quarter-mile hike and those bags are heavy. Anyway, I'll have to rouse George. You go banging around, he'll figure some drunk's trying to give him a bad time. He knows my voice."

I was grateful for Slim. It was all I could do to plod through the puddles without the weight of a bag. George's house was dark. Slim pounded on the door and swore with a mighty voice. From inside came an answering voice, thick with sleep.

"Dammit, Slim! Don't break the door down. I'm coming. Hell of a night you pick to bring me guests." But he was not angry. He had donned a rain slicker, boots, and a hat to escort us next door to the hotel. "You must be a mite tired," he said kindly.

I was, and as I stretched out on the bed some minutes later and thought back on that long day, I knew why so few braved the west coast.

January 1, 1960. A beautiful clear cold day had followed the stormy night. We dressed slowly, speculating on whether Bill had received our radiogram. After a leisurely breakfast we strolled down to the dock. To our surprise, Bill was already there with his wife, Joan, and Vicki. She sprang into Wally's arms, yipping her delight.

"Son of a gun!" Wally exclaimed, stroking Vicki's back. "You missed us, eh?"

A ten-minute flight now became an hour-and-a-half excursion. I had never really appreciated the twists and turns of the channel, the hidden nooks, the silver streams flowing into the salt. We had passed over too quickly.

"Maybe you'd like to ride with us when we go in for mail and supplies," Bill suggested.

"We would," Wally agreed. "Sure you won't mind stopping by?"

"Hell, no. It's not out of the way."

We were home at last.

Chapter 31

Winter winds raged, and the rains came. We raced to the beach to watch, laughing and shouting in a delirium of exhilaration. If this was a lonely life, in this tiny world of our own, we were unaware of it.

On the twenty-second of January I would celebrate my birthday. For a full week before, the old house was charged with secrecy. Every night I was sent to bed early. Lying there, listening to Wally's happy whistle, it was hard to concentrate on my book. In a mischievous mood, I'd call down to him. His cheerful answer was mildly threatening.

"Don't you dare come down."

He served me my birthday breakfast in bed. Then I followed him down the stairs and there were my gifts. Four cracker tins had been transformed into a canister set, their original purpose concealed by a coat of pink paint. A breadboard leaned against the canisters. The sea, an unwitting participant in this game of surprises, had floated in the perfect board for loving hands to sand and resand to the exact degree of smoothness. A third gift was a wastebasket, also painted pink. Such a lump rose in my throat that it almost choked back the words.

"They're beautiful!"

"Good thing I bought plenty of pink when we painted the kitchen," Wally commented. "I intended buying you a present in town, but with this weather I knew Joan and Bill would never make it over."

"And I'm glad. These are the best gifts ever."

The storms continued but it didn't matter that the winds growled and the rains rushed down. We had time, that most precious of gifts, and we treasured each moment. Finally the rains did stop and we had a visitor. It was the second of February. Long before a boat could be sighted, we had picked up the hum of an engine. It had to be *Maggie*.

"Want to go to town?" Bill shouted.

We launched our skiff and rowed out. Bill gave us a hand aboard, and we set out, our skiff bouncing merrily in *Maggie*'s wake.

The air was crystal.

Near Zeballos the water had a greenish cast and patches of white, soft and mushy, pushed against us. Bill slowed to a snail's pace, knowing that only the surface was mushy, that beneath were razor-edged chunks of ice. Getting to Zeballos had seemed incidental, but now that it was within sight our interest quickened. Zeballos had mail, and supplies for us.

But Bill shook his head. "Can't make it," he said.

As we backed off we saw the RCMP boat approaching. Her steel prow cut through the ice, her backwash forcing the ice patches aside.

After a month of isolation, a day in town was an occasion. We chatted with friends, bought everything we could think of, ate dinner at the café—such a treat to eat out! We collected our mail, a sackful, letters and cards and mysterious packages. In late afternoon, staggering under the burden of our loot, we returned to *Maggie*.

The slow cruise home was a perfect ending to a magnificent day. Over our shoulders a silvery moon glided serenely into position above the snowcapped peaks, silently competing with the rosy glow of the setting sun as it dipped over the horizon.

February was a singularly delightful month. The high-pitched whine of *Maggie*'s engine sent us racing to the beach. Soothed by *Maggie*'s gentle sideways rock as she wallowed in the troughs, we roved aimlessly, returning home only when darkness threatened to engulf us.

Too soon, February gave way to March and the return of

the rains. Many days still centered around *Maggie*, but our voyages now had purpose and destination. The ice at the heads of the inlets, impervious to the rays of the sun, now gave way to the gentle persistence of the rain. Access to Zeballos brought renewed demand for our services. Our labors depended on Bill's cooperation and *Maggie*'s dependability, but *Maggie* was reliable, and Bill, easygoing and good-natured, never complained about the frequency of the trips or the time involved.

One old springer was of special concern. He was old and tired, and pressed against our legs, soft brown eyes beseeching.

"Dammit, Hank!" Wally said. "I'd do anything for the old fellow, but no matter what I do, it's only a matter of time."

"I know." There was resignation in Hank's voice. "Best damn friend I ever had. That tumor on his front leg is so painful."

"I can remove it, Hank, but I'm certain it's cancerous."

"If it makes him easier even for a little while, it's worth it."

Wally shook his head. "Awful risk! The old heart is barely making it. He could kick out right while we're operating."

"Do it, Doc!" It was an order.

I knew how to hold the legs between my fingers while Wally administered the ether. When the breathing was normal I took the ether cone, still restraining the back legs with my left hand. I checked respiration, the eyes, the color of the tongue, alert for any sign the heart wouldn't take it. Suddenly the old body lurched convulsively. The hind legs jerked as if released by a spring. I felt my wrist snap.

"God! We've got to finish," Wally exhorted. "He's still going. Use your elbow. Keep those legs out of my way."

It was done. The old dog roused from the ether groggy, disoriented, but with the love in his eyes shining through. Hank knelt beside him, making no attempt now to hide the tears in his eyes.

"Gad, you old son of a gun, you made it!" He ran a gentle hand down the emaciated body, then buried his face in the shaggy coat. Wally motioned to me, and we left them alone.

"I knew you broke it," Wally ranted as he examined my wrist, "but I kept telling myself it couldn't be. Well, it's a nice clean break, but for God's sake, try to keep out of trouble till it mends."

There was no time to dwell on my plight. One of our dreams had been to have our furniture shipped up from Seattle. It would be unloaded at Esperanza, and Bill and several of the Indians had agreed to cart it on out to the cove.

The day the furniture was to arrive, April winds howled and the rain was heavy. Our freight would be dumped regardless. The small shed at Esperanza could never accommodate so many crates. Bill knew. He stopped by only long enough to reassure us.

"Gathered up some waterproof tarps, Doc. I'll fix 'em."

It was several days before the rains stopped, but then Bill appeared, trailed by two trollers. It would have to be high tide for the trollers to return and enter our cove, yet every throb of an engine sent us scurrying to the beach. When at last they came, my eyes widened at the assortment of crates stacked high on their decks.

"Do we own all that?"

"Afraid so!" Wally's voice held a kind of awe.

One by one, the trollers edged past our reefs. Skiffs were lowered, crates ripped apart to reduce weight.

Once the troller was unloaded, others packed up what they could, but no one worked harder than Wally. He never slackened. I watched him and worried that he seemed so tired.

"Fix us some supper, Chicken," he said.

The house was a shambles, but everything we owned was there. The men sat at the table, digging hungrily at the food, slurping up cup after cup of coffee. It was over and we had done it.

Chapter 32

Spring brought a certain loveliness to our cove: sights and sounds and smells of new life everywhere. However, all Vancouver Island had been deluged with mice, and we did not suffer alone. A logging camp boasted they had disposed of one hundred and eighty of the pests in one night. Someone must have counted them with fiendish delight.

"Can't we do something?" I demanded of Wally.

He'd always been able to contrive whatever was needed. Surely his inventive ability wouldn't fail us now. He set me to poking through the garbage for an empty milk tin, and he disappeared into the woodshed. He returned with a length of fine wire and a discarded five-gallon can. I watched curiously as he punched two holes, across from each other, near the top of the can. Next he took the milk tin, punching holes in the exact center, top and bottom. He passed the wire through these holes, then the holes in the can, securing the ends of the wire so the milk tin hung taut over the can. A slat from the woodshed provided an adequate ramp.

"Let's have some of that cheese spread you've been hoarding," he said.

It was expensive, but I didn't wince as he generously coated all sides of the milk tin. The slat was placed just far enough from the tin so that a hungry mouse must stretch or jump to get at the cheese. Either movement would set the tin spinning, sending an unwary mouse to the bottom of the can. We poured water in to a depth of five inches and sat back to await our first victim. We didn't wait long. Splashings occurred with increasing frequency, and I gloated without shame over each fatal plunge. Not so, Wally! Had I not resisted his inclination, I'm certain he'd have discarded the trap.

"Poor little devil," he'd sigh as the splashing became frantic. "I'd better dispatch him and put him out of his misery."

Though the mice were an aggravation, they could not thwart the miracle of spring. We had planted our garden. Tiny shoots, eager for the light, stirred the sod with restless determination. Bees tested each fragile blossom, and birds filled the air with their songs of gladness. Minniebelle returned, taking up a position in the salmonberry bushes at our kitchen window. We wondered at her audacity. We could almost have reached out and touched her, but she regarded us passively, her head cocked at an impertinent angle.

As we sat there, watching and marveling, Wally fashioned stories he hoped to write. "Tales of the Nootka Woods," he called them. Minniebelle, of course, was the heroine. Certainly it would be hard to ignore this one who persistently guarded our window. Though her actions aroused our curiosity, we didn't pry. Later we were glad we'd refrained.

Wally spotted the miracle first. "Look!" he cried, his voice trembling with excitement. "Minniebelle has babies."

Proudly, unafraid, Minniebelle marched her progeny down the path, past the kitchen door, at our very feet, and, clucking instructions, led them straight to the garden.

"Look at that!" Wally exclaimed. "Minniebelle the grouse-mother showing her kids through the garden, telling them, 'This is the lettuce, these are the onions, here is the parsley.'"
In a hushed voice he marveled at her wisdom. I knew in a flash we would share that garden and that our share might be small, but who could resist those shrill peeps or Minniebelle's maternal clucks!

One day as I was thinning the brush along the kitchen path, I made a discovery that eloquently revealed Minniebelle's reason for maintaining, those earlier weeks, her faithful stance at our window. Concealed in the brush lay the broken shells of her brood. Instinct had prompted her to make her nest in as close proximity to man as was possible. Here her babies had been safe from her natural enemies, who were unlikely to venture so near. If they did, we would see and defend her. Quite deliberately, she had sought us out.

This episode with Minniebelle added impetus to Wally's stories. But he seemed reluctant to put them on paper. I wished he would. On dull rainy days when it was more pleasurable to be inside than out, I, too, had an urge to write. Contrarily, he seemed to resent it. He said nothing, but if I took pen in hand, a slight frown and a certain impatience discouraged me. One gloomy day, having pushed my writing aside so as not to displease him, I decided I must know his reason.

"I thought we'd both planned to write," I said. "But whenever you see me with a pen it seems to upset you. Don't you want me to?"

"Of course I want you to, but not now. Now we must talk. You can write later."

"But when?" I persisted.

"The time will come."

I cheated occasionally, jotting down notes, yet avoided any open endeavor. Other matters were more pressing. Getting water to the house was a primary concern.

"Gravity's our best bet, I think," Wally said. "We can build a damn in the creek above the waterfall and use plastic hose to bring the water to the house. Let's measure how much hose we'll need."

We struggled through the tangled brush along the shore and up the steep sides of the waterfall, plotting our course with dogged determination. A thousand feet to reach the proposed site of our dam. It was staggering, but Wally was undaunted.

"So be it. We'll get an order off to Simpson Sears in Vancouver, and while we're waiting we'll take a run down to Seattle."

"What do you mean, a run?" I groaned, remembering that long, long trip in December.

"Whatever! We've got to get the pigeon back. Can't expect Bill to keep running errands for us now fishing's started. Then there's Alaska and . . ." He paused dramatically. "I figure it's about time we looked into buying the cottage."

"You mean it!"

"Yep! We still want it, don't we? When Bill comes in we'll get him to run us to Zeballos. Maybe we'll fly out with B.C. Airlines. No weather problems now. No loitering in Seattle, though. We'll pick up the pigeon and come right back."

I knew he wouldn't be able to resist a peek at Greg, but it was hardly more than a hello and a good-bye. In a sense, I felt cheated . . . until we stopped at Esperanza to see Dr. McLean. It was so easy. He actually wanted to sell. So at last that lovely little cottage was ours, along with 116 acres of timber.

There was no time to make plans for the cottage. There were calls in Zeballos and Tahsis and Tofino and preparations for our northern clinics. Our hose hadn't arrived, but there would have been no time to lay it. Bill promised to pick it up on one of his runs to Zeballos.

Dew lay heavy on the grass the morning of the day we set to fly north, and though the sun was already high in the sky, there was a decided chill. Zeballos looked like such a sleepy, peaceful little town it seemed a shame to disturb it, but the roar of our engine, reverberating against the mountain peaks, was a guaranteed awakener. Howie Sutton tried to get us a weather report, but the mysterious elements that make up our atmosphere blocked every attempt. We shrugged it off. With skies so blue, how could the weather not be good?

As we approached Tahsis, Wally set the pigeon in a climb to carry us over the top of the mountains and into the central valley of Vancouver Island. It was like flying into a bed of cotton tufts. Clouds swirled about our wing tips, forcing us lower and lower, and out over the Strait a gray mass obscured all but a rim of the sea. Then the fog engulfed us, gray sky blending with the water. How many times we had groped our way to Sullivan Bay. Instinct alone could have guided us. The Germaines, who had taken over for the Collinsons, heard the drone of our engine, not too surprised at all that we should appear out of the mists.

Out of Bella Bella the next morning, fog again overtook us. At Wright Sound five channels branch out in sundry directions, a confusing hodgepodge at any time. Now, with fog swirling in from the sea, it was completely indecipherable.

"Well, Chicken, I guess we set down."

"I guess," I replied.

Then the fog lifted, not even to treetop level, but enough so that we tentatively identified the channel we sought. Wally swung the pigeon in that direction, then gave a whoop of joy. A troller, appearing out of the mists, chugged slowly by us.

"That troller can't be going anywhere but to Prince Rupert!"

We circled back, took a heading off the troller, and were on our way. In the narrow confines of Grenville Channel it would be virtually impossible to stray.

This trip was like any other, and yet, inexplicably, it was different. "We won't hurry," Wally kept reiterating. "We won't leave until we've seen everyone who wants to see us."

We worked at a more leisurely pace. Even our shop had not required too much effort. Wally was in a reflective mood, unusual for him, for he was more wont to look ahead than back.

"Herb was right," he said. "We've never wanted for a place to set up our clinic."

"Agreed," I admitted, "though I thought we'd never get the grease and grime scrubbed from the walls of that little café."

"It was bad. My favorite, though, was the Bon Marché basement, even carrying the water. Amazing none of the customers in the store upstairs complained."

"I liked the fur shop best," I reminisced. "That huge plate glass window let in so much light."

"Ah! You just enjoyed the attention we got there."

Certainly we'd had no privacy. The shop was located on the

main street facing the docks. Tourists from the steamers had vied with the local citizenry for a vantage point at our window. For Wally this was no distraction. He concentrated on his work, oblivious to all else. Not I! I'd been unable to resist an occasional swift glance to ascertain the size of our audience.

Our reminiscing was cut short as Al Baker walked into the clinic. "Knock it off early tonight, folks. Fran and I want you to come to dinner. I'll pick you up about seven."

Brownie met us at the door when Al drove us over that evening. She was an older Brownie than the one that had waggled from end to end when Al had brought her to us as a three-month-old puppy, but she still waggled, and begged for attention.

"Al," Wally said, stroking her head, "you've got the healthiest dog in Ketchikan, I do believe."

"She's had a good doctor."

"Maybe! But a lot of the credit goes to you. You kept her trim after we spayed her. Makes a man feel good when he sees someone has really followed directions. Yep, Brownie," he said, bending to scratch her ears, "you are a good girl, all right."

We had time for clients, and time for friends. We followed the same pattern in Prince Rupert, determined that no one who wished to see us would be disappointed.

"Do you realize we're losing money on this trip?" I asked Wally.

He seemed bent on giving his services away, holding fees at a minimum. He looked at me thoughtfully, not denying the charge. When he spoke his words were a gentle reproof.

"Aren't you glad we can afford to lose money?"

It was more a statement of fact than a question, and I felt a quick sense of shame, realizing that the love and respect of these people was the pay that counted. In Wally they had found a man of rare understanding, a man never too busy or weary to hear them out. How many times he had said, "We have two patients, the animal and the owner. You can't treat one without treating the other."

Those were wonderful days in Prince Rupert. We had dinner with Viv and visited with Lucy. I took no notice that Wally was tired.

We were homebound at last. Spotty weather reports had not been encouraging, so fog patches were no surprise. If there was fog anywhere along our route, we could expect to find it in the Bella Bella area.

There was no dismay at being forced to make a stop. Taxiing up to the dock at Bella Bella rekindled memories of past years when that stop had been a must. We were secretly grateful that the fog, which for years had teased and tormented us, had forced us once again to seek shelter with old friends. We responded to the warmth from the cookstove in the Tites' cheerful kitchen, our conversation interrupted, as before, by the persistent blare of the radio. It seemed appropriate, on this particular journey, when we had made such a special effort to see all the friends won over a period of years, that the agenda should include a stay with the Tites.

We stopped at Sullivan Bay briefly, since home was an hour's flight farther on. Already we anticipated the blue waters of Esperanza Inlet, deepening to dark green in the shadow of our cove. What a fitting finale, that flight across the forested expanse of Vancouver Island, the snowcapped peaks of the west coast beckoning, the soft breezes wafting our pigeon up and over the heights until, with startling abruptness, the mountains gave way and the blue Pacific stretched before us.

Chapter 33

We strolled the beaches and poked about our cottage. There was much work to be done! Our days were haphazard, regulated only by the sun and the tides. Supper waited while the vivid colors in the evening sky deepened, blending with the black of night. The nights, too, had significance, the nocturnal sky a colossal stage featuring magnificent heavenly displays. No fog crept in to dim the brilliance of the aurora borealis flooding our skies, lavishing upon our small domain an eerie light that enabled us to walk fearlessly over the rocks.

We could have just drifted along with these miracles had it not been for a quick trip to Zeballos and a letter from Maureen. Dick would be at Army Reserve camp for two weeks, and she wanted to come up with Greg. In my mind's eye I saw water for formulas, water for baths, and an endless supply of diapers.

The hose for our water supply had to be unrolled. Hose that has been snugged into rolls does not give any indication it will ever lie flat. Like an ugly black snake, it writhed and coiled, fighting us every step of the way. We reached the waterfall, scratched from thorny encounters with berry bushes, our clothing torn, our hair a tangle of leaves and twigs.

"I feel like I've been through a war," I groaned. "We'll never make it to the top of the waterfall."

"We will," Wally assured me. "It'll be easier now."

He was right. The brush actually assisted. Firmly rooted

to either bank, it provided handholds on our climb to the top. Exhausted, we flopped to the ground, but the obstinate hose lay in place.

"Enough for today," Wally decreed. "We'll fix the water box tomorrow."

Our box had slats on two sides. Wally covered the bottom and sides with a fine mesh screen to keep out silt. In one end he drilled a hole, the exact circumference of the hose. We placed our box in a quiet pool about a hundred feet back from the top of the falls, securing it with boulders. Now the hose must be shoved through the hole. Wally's muscles quivered, his face reddened with the exertion, but the hose resisted.

"Can't we make the hole larger?" I protested. "I don't like you straining like that."

"It has to fit or it's no damn good. There! It's in!"

A heavy sigh escaped him, and I knew a vague uneasiness. The effort had been too great. But he insisted on going ahead with the dam, and I helped. It was a crude affair, a large plank across the stream, reinforced with rocks and mud and moss, but it worked. We watched, jubilant, as the water level rose in our box.

Back at the house, gleaming new faucets were installed over the kitchen sink with their proper intake and outlet hoses. To me, it all seemed so complicated, but Wally worked with assurance.

"Turn on the faucet, Chicken," he said when he was finished.

The faucet felt cold and smooth in my hand. I pulled the lever forward, and a stream of clear cold water flowed into our sink. How many times, those next few days, we turned on the faucet just to witness again that flow of clear cold water!

That afternoon Paul Smith came in from Nuchatlitz. "Want to buy a boat, Doc? My boat goes faster than yours. I need money."

Wally's eyes twinkled. "Why not? We'll need it," he said to me by way of explanation, "to haul Maureen and Greg around."

I had to laugh. "We sure make up our minds in a hurry."

"Run me home, Doc," Paul proposed. "Then it's yours."

Everything we did was focused around Greg's needs. In our tiniest bedroom a cot was embraced by three walls. On the beach lay a sheet of plywood that had floated in one day. It couldn't have been cut better to size, fitting perfectly from wall to wall on the exposed side of the cot. With hooks at either end, it made a satisfactory enclosure. To my mind it seemed we'd anticipated every need.

Wally had an inspiration: Greg should have a swing. It had to be a very special swing, one that would hold a small boy safely and swing with no effort.

"I have it," he said finally. "Let's put that boat to good use. I can get what I need at Queens Cove."

Maureen and Greg were traveling via the *Tahsis Prince*, which, in addition to freight, had accommodations for eight passengers. After a three-day voyage from Vancouver, they were scheduled to arrive in Zeballos late in the afternoon of August 14.

"Let's pick them up in Esperanza," Wally suggested. "No sense in their going on to Zeballos."

Long before the scheduled arrival, we took our stand on the dock, waiting for the first glimpse of the freighter as she steamed through the Tahsis Narrows. At last! She inched up to the tiny dock. I waited impatiently while a sling was loaded with crates and lifted up and over the side of the ship, coming to rest almost at my feet.

"Could I come aboard?" I called up to the captain. "My daughter's there somewhere."

"Sure! Hop on that sling there and hang on."

I looked at Wally. His grin was a challenge. Resolutely, I stepped onto the sling, grasped the ropes with tight fists, and was swung high into the air, up and over, then dumped unceremoniously at the bottom of the hold, along with boxes of outgoing freight.

"I'll take you up to the dining room," one of the deckhands said to me. "The passengers are at dinner."

I stopped at the door. Greg sat at the head of the table, the center of attention. Maureen looked up, saw me, and gasped.

"Mother! Where did you come from?"

"I came aboard with the freight. Saves a lot of time picking you up here."

She gathered her things together while I bundled up Greg. The captain lowered the gangplank, and I carried my wiggling bundle to Wally's waiting arms. Maureen followed with her bags. The remaining passengers had deserted the dining room. For all of them, it was a first trip into bush country. As we laid Greg on the dock and wrapped him in a life jacket, bits of their conversation floated down to us.

"They must be out of their minds."

One woman called down to Maureen, "How can you take a baby out on the sea in such a small boat? Aren't you terrified?"

Maureen laughed, shaking her head. Then she climbed into our new speedboat and Wally pulled away from the dock, away from the freighter with its incredulous passengers.

The sea was choppy and our boat slapped rhythmically, but no one minded, least of all Greg. He sat on my lap, his eyes big with wonder, gurgling with delight, but he sat very still, seeming to sense in his little one-year-old mind that this was no time to be wriggling around.

Greg took to the cove as if he'd been raised there, paddling contentedly at the tide line, with one of us hovering near to be certain his adventuresome spirit didn't entice him too far. He crawled along the beach, unmindful of the rocks, until the toes of his tiny shoes were scuffed through and the knees of his little trousers hung in shreds. When rain forced us to remain indoors, he sat in his swing, shouting gleefully.

Maureen swam in the clear green water of the cove, rowed out to the rougher water beyond, explored our islands, our beaches, happy and carefree with Greg in our hands. These were times that Wally treasured.

Two weeks had gone by, and they had to return to Seattle.

We took them to Zeballos, and on our way home I sat immersed in my own private gloom. Then I heard Wally sigh.

He looked terribly tired. In the excitement of the past two weeks I'd taken no notice. I'd make it up to him, I vowed. For the moment, I simply squeezed his arm, that he might know I was glad to be alone with him.

Chapter 34

Our work schedule had been published in the *Ketchikan Daily News*, our hotel reservations were in order, but I sensed in Wally a vague reluctance to set out. I didn't press him. After the excitement of the past two weeks, these lazy days together were precious.

"They've waited on us before in Ketchikan." Then I giggled. "But this is the first time we haven't flown because the weather is too nice."

As the days passed, days perfect for flying, and he still gave no indication of wanting to leave, I became puzzled. To pass up such weather at this time of the year was tempting the fates.

Thinking to prod him into action, I suggested, "How about flying up to Zeballos to pick up the mail?"

"Oh, I don't know. It's so lovely here. I hate to miss a minute of it."

There was a sadness in his voice that disturbed me. Why, when the world was so beautiful, should he be sad? Did he not want to go to Alaska? Why did he object even to a short hop to Zeballos?

The following day I observed again that inexpressible sadness. There was a faraway look in his eyes that seemed to exclude me.

"What is it?" I asked. "This has been the most wonderful summer, yet you seem almost unhappy. I don't understand it."

He hesitated a moment. "It's just that there's so much I've wanted to do and I feel I've accomplished so little."

"How can you say such a thing?" I protested. "Who else would have taken on a practice like ours? And look at all we've done here. Take a look at those roses. To coax our rocky soil to produce beauty like that to me is the most remarkable achievement of all."

He smiled, and a little of the sadness left his eyes. "You think I've done all right then?"

"I most certainly do. Anyway, we have all our lives. One thing at a time! It will all get done."

"I've often wondered," he mused, "how a person could enjoy a place like this, like the Newtons, knowing they'd never see the completion of their plans." He paused, searching for an answer. "I guess true happiness lies in the doing, not in the completion. Reminds me of the story of the three priests who were told they had but an hour to live and each, in turn, was asked how he'd spend that hour. One replied he would spend it in prayer. The second decided he would hasten to visit his mother, but the third said he would go along as usual, giving his best to every single minute. I think," he concluded, "that is the only answer."

"Of course it's the answer."

The serious mood seemed to have passed. I was relieved, yet in the back of my mind, his mood and the words he had spoken troubled me.

That evening as we walked hand in hand along the beach, a sudden dazzling display of northern lights held us spellbound. There were no flashes of light appearing, disappearing, and reappearing. A glittering arc hung stationary in the night sky, as if held by some unspeakable power. Then, as suddenly as it had come, it vanished.

A glorious day followed that night of splendor, but there was that aura of sadness I couldn't explain, couldn't wish away.

That night I had a dream. I saw our cove, the beautiful blue sky, the green waters: so still, so serene. Suddenly a churning black cloud appeared, blotting out the blue skies.

The waters of the cove turned inky black, burbling wickedly along the shoreline in thousands of miniature caldrons. Off to one side, six figures sat on a log, their backs to me. In the next instant, a seaplane swooped down on the cove and pulled up to the shore. The door was flung open, revealing three figures in white. One of them motioned with a finger. Five figures on the log remained immobile, but one turned and, responding to that beckoning finger, ran straight to the plane and was pulled inside. The door slammed shut and the plane soared into the heavens, now again miraculously blue.

At this point I awoke, shaking with terror. Wally was not in bed. I ran down the stairs to the kitchen.

"I couldn't sleep," he mumbled. "But I'll sleep now."

He sat in his chair by the kitchen window, arms folded on the table, his head resting on his arms, and he did sleep, but even in sleep he looked so unutterably weary. Many times he had slept like this, catnaps that refreshed him, but this sleep was different. Distraught and uneasy, I wandered down to the beach. Vicki watched me go, not offering to come. Usually she loved to romp on the beach. This time she refused to leave the side of her master.

Our glorious weather had vanished. The skies were gray, and the wind tossed the waves in disdainful black curls. I fought a feeling of hopelessness, my every instinct crying out for help. Back to the house I went, propelled more by impulse than deliberation. Wally was still asleep. The feeling we needed help persisted. Perhaps if I hung a towel from the branch of a tree, a passing boat might see it and come in. I stood there on the beach a long time, watching the towel whip in the wind. And no boat came.

When I returned to the house Wally was awake, not wanting to talk, still wanting me there. Before he drifted off again he looked at me, a long moment. When he spoke, his voice was so low I barely heard the words. "You will scream and cry, but you will be all right."

What could he mean? Why was I so afraid? Restless, I

sought the beach with a vain hope, for it was now past six.
As I stood there, an animal emerged from the trees on the
far side of the cove. My eyes followed its movements, and
as it came nearer I saw it was a black bear.

A bear right on our own beach! "Wally will never believe
this," I thought. "I'll take a picture, or if he's awake, I'll tell
him."

But Wally was asleep. What a pity! He'd want to see our
bear. Well, all the more reason for a picture. I sped to the
beach, my fears forgotten. The bear ambled in my direction,
stopping now and again to lift a boulder and send it crashing
against the rocks. This was a hungry bear, no mistake, in
search of clams and other edible sea life. He indicated no
interest in me other than to look up occasionally, his great head
swinging from side to side. Emboldened by his indifference, I
sauntered toward him. He looked up, inspecting me curiously,
but made no motion to leave. I stood my ground and took
my picture. In fact, I took several, and retreated to the house in
triumph. If only Wally would waken.

I kept the fire going and got a blanket to cover Wally with.
At last, weary with watching, I lay down on the davenport. If
he stirred, I would hear him.

I dozed fitfully. Then, abruptly, I was wide awake. Vicki
was whining, and I could hear the scurry of her feet, as if she
were running in circles. I ran to the kitchen. Wally lay sprawled
facedown on the floor. Shaking with dread, I knelt beside
him. I knew he was dead, but it couldn't be. I reached out a
hand to touch him, and then I did as he had foretold. I
screamed and cried.

"How could you?" I cried. "How could you go and leave me
alone?"

It was one o'clock in the morning of the fifth of September,
and I was alone except for Vicki. She whined and pushed at
my arm, but it gave me no comfort. I sat through the long
night, dreading the day I could not escape, reminding myself
that I must not panic. Wally would not have wanted me to
panic.

I needed help and couldn't just wait for someone to stop in. Everyone who knew about our Alaska schedule probably thought we'd already left.

The storm was over. The skies were blue. Boats should be passing. Once Father Lobsinger had advised us, "If ever you're in trouble, hang out a sheet as a signal."

"Vicki," I ordered, "watch him. Keep the mice away."

Stripping both sheets from the bed, I ran to the farthest point of the beach and climbed up a ledge. I had to stretch to reach the branches of a stunted tree fighting for a foothold in the rock, but I succeeded in securing the sheet at the two opposite corners.

Now the other sheet. The tide was low. I could wade to our islands and climb to the highest point.

I waited a long time and finally heard both a boat and a plane. I ran to the beach, ripped the towel from the branches where it had hung all the night, and waved it madly, shouting at the top of my lungs. I seized a rusty rod lying on the beach and beat on a pan, but the low-flying plane gave no indication I'd been seen and the boat passed on by. With a heavy heart, I returned to the house.

My eyes focused on our radiophone. Our morning schedule came over the air at 10:20. The phone had been a contact we'd not needed, but had enjoyed. We'd answered our calls, but seldom sent messages. The phone had been Wally's concern.

"I wish you'd learn to use this thing," he'd told me more than once, almost crossly. "Someday you'll be sorry."

"Okay," I'd said, but I'd not paid attention. As I looked at our radio now, properly disconnected to conserve the battery, I was sorry! I didn't know positive from negative or one wire from another, but somehow I must make it work. I made connections, my fingers trembling, and I turned various switches, as I'd seen Wally do, but no voices came. Then I remembered it was Labor Day. Perhaps no one would be on.

"Stoltz Logging . . . Flynn's Camp calling Green Logging . . . Flynn's Camp calling Esperanza . . . Zeballos . . ."

Over and over, but not one answer. Was it because no one

was listening, or had I failed to make the proper connections? Hysteria choked my voice "Please! Does anybody hear me? I need help."

Then there was a voice. "Spring Island answering. Go ahead."

The words tumbled out. "This is Flynn's Camp. Dr. Flynn is dead. It was a heart attack, I think. I'm all alone. I don't know what to do."

The voice was calm. "I'll take over. Turn off your set, and don't worry. I'll stay on the air until I contact someone."

Spring Island was a weather station thirty miles to the north, and not on our schedule. How had they happened to be listening? But it didn't matter. I dropped onto my knees beside Vicki.

"Someone will come, Vicki. Someone will!"

I picked up the Bible, letting it fall open, and read at random. I listened, and I ran to the beach innumerable times, imagining I heard the whine of an engine. I saw my bear, but I ignored it.

It was two o'clock in the afternoon when I did hear a boat. A skiff was lowered, and Mrs. McLean rowed in to shore.

"We came as soon as we heard," she said, putting her arms around me.

Then came the RCMP boat. They took Wally to Esperanza, and I followed with Mrs. McLean. Mr. Pettersen came to take me to Tahsis, where there was a telephone. I called Maureen. I called Pop Flynn. I even called Ketchikan to notify them we wouldn't be coming as scheduled. "Bring him home," Pop said.

How long that night was! I tossed and turned in the strange bed, crying out against my aloneness, and Mrs. McLean was unable to comfort me. In the morning Mr. Pettersen came again, this time to take me to Zeballos to arrange for transportation, for Wally and for myself. I listened stonily as Howie explained that a plane would fly us to Port Alberni, that a mortician would meet us.

"I'm sorry," he said. "There has to be an autopsy. It's international law. I've reserved you a room." He paused and brushed a hand across his eyes.

I followed Mr. Pettersen back to the boat. I sat stiff and unapproachable, and I cried. Mr. Pettersen leaned toward me and put a hand on my shoulder.

"You shouldn't cry. Doc wouldn't want you to cry. He isn't very far away. He wouldn't go too far from you. He loved you too much." Simple words, but the tears ceased. I didn't have to wait long at Esperanza for the plane.

"It's okay," the pilot said. I climbed in.

And so we were flying once more, Wally and I, over those mountains we both loved.

It was the day before Christmas, and I realized that it was twelve years since we'd been married. I was at Maureen's and Dick's when a package came for me from Prince Rupert. I removed the wrappings, and there was the etching of the bear and the salmon that I had so admired and wanted on our last trip to Prince Rupert.

Wally had known he was sick. Why hadn't he told me? Perhaps he had, in many ways, but I hadn't seen because I couldn't conceive of life without him.

BOOK TWO

A Place of
Refuge

Chapter 35

My eyes followed the upward, outward flight of the little seaplane until it was lost to me beyond the horizon. For the present, at least, my sole contact with the world had vanished. I stood as if rooted to the rocks that converged along the shoreline. My mind raced back to the farewell party in Seattle that had been given in my honor so few days ago.

"Nootka Island!" someone had questioned. "Never heard of it. Where is it anyway?"

"Of course you've heard of it," I'd retorted. "That's where Wally and I were living when he died last September."

"Bethine Flynn! You're not going back there? Not alone? A half-pint like you!" There was horror in her voice. "No roads, no phones, no neighbors! Going with Wally was one thing, but by yourself, and at your age, a grandmother!"

"Oh, come on!" I protested. "You make me sound positively ancient. My grandson isn't even two years old yet. Besides, I like it there."

"Oh, sure! When you're down here! But wait until you get there and there isn't a soul you can turn to."

"Don't worry." Another woman spoke, laughter tinkling in her voice. "This isn't good-bye. We'll see you next week."

Off in the distance now a fishing troller edged along Center Island, the muted throb of its motor somehow harmonizing with the tranquility that surrounded me. I watched idly, knowing it would not come near, for no one was aware of my presence.

As I watched, the thought processes of my mind pushed me further into the past, back to the day when Wally and I, together, had discovered this paradise and loved it. This cove on Nootka Island, two hundred miles northwest of Victoria, on Vancouver Island's forbidding west coast, had satisfied our longings. It was the beauty we loved, the isolation we craved, a retreat from the pressures of a busy schedule.

But what about now? Would I again find it a place of refuge, or would I be held, like a prisoner, unable to escape those memories of past years? Would I be able to appreciate the quiet beauty of this lonely place? I had to know. Wally's words, not too long before he died, came back to me now.

"If anything should happen to me, would you try to live here?"

I was here. I picked up my bags and trudged determinedly along the rocky shore and up the steps that led to the old log house.

As I took the last step, there was a rustle in the huckleberry bushes. Minniebelle the grouse mother emerged and strutted down the path ahead of me . . . a few running steps, then slow, deliberate steps, cocking her head from side to side as if saying, "It's about time you got here." Then, with a swirl of wings, she came to rest in the old plum tree, from which she regarded me silently.

"Minniebelle, you rascal!" I exclaimed. "How nice of you to be here to welcome me."

I smiled as she pecked at the still-green plums. How completely she had taken over this place! My eyes strayed to the house, a two-story structure, seven rooms in all, grayed by many summers, but sturdy still. At the peak of the roof, beneath the overhang of the shakes, "1914" had been inscribed in bold letters. The house had weathered almost half a century.

Everything was as I had left it . . . with one exception. Buckets I had set out to catch the drips from the kitchen roof in heavy rains were now filled with water and worse. Tiny grotesque bodies were floating on the surface—unwary mice, killed by their own curiosity.

I shuddered and grimaced, repelled by the smell of dead mice, thankful nonetheless that they were dead. "Darn leaky roof!" I muttered.

I remembered the last time I'd been here. It was in early January, after the long trip by bus from Maureen's home in Seattle, across the Washington–British Columbia border to Vancouver, then by ferry to Nanaimo on Vancouver Island's east coast, and again by bus, eighty miles north and sixty miles west, to the Gold River logging camp on the west coast of the island, the end of the road. From Gold River all travel was by boat or by seaplane.

It was dark and snowing hard when I boarded the *Uchuck*, the small passenger and freight ship that serviced our isolated west coast area. The wind shrieked up Muchalot Inlet, our ship protesting the chop of the sea. I sat staring at an empty window, for the black of night had erased all the world. I felt lost and lonely and wondered whether, in such a storm, Greg, a neighbor, would be able to make it to the mission hospital at Esperanza, where he was to pick me up.

"Excuse me," said a voice at my elbow. "Mrs. Flynn, isn't it?"

"Johnny Schoppel! Oh, you don't know how good it is to see someone I know."

Johnny Schoppel operated an independent logging operation in Tahsis Inlet. He and his wife, Crystal, had visited Wally and me at the cove. I poured out my worries to him now.

"Well now, I'm glad I spotted you. Greg's been working at my place this last week. He'll still be there. You get off with me and spend the night with us. Greg can take you on in the morning."

"Thank you, but I really couldn't. It's so late, and Crystal isn't expecting me. I wouldn't want to put her to a lot of bother."

"Nonsense! She'll be glad to have you. Besides, it'll be midnight before this ship makes it to Esperanza. We're bucking a heavy wind."

"Well . . ." I hesitated.

"No wells! You'll be doing me a favor. I've been to town, you know. Meant to pick up a box of chocolates or a dozen roses for the wife. It's our anniversary today. But I forgot. Hate to come home empty-handed. You'll be a nice surprise."

I was a surprise. Crystal had turned on the dock lights and rushed out to meet Johnny. He ignored her, concerned with assisting me down the ladder from the deck of the *Uchuck* to the swaying dock, but from my place on the ladder, pressed hard against the ship's hull, I could see her hesitation. One thing was evident—I was not the surprise she'd expected.

"Crystal!" Johnny called out. "I brought you a surprise. I brought you Mrs. Flynn."

She recovered quickly. "How nice! Come in out of this awful weather."

Their camp was built on a series of floats, which facilitated moving the camp to another location when the logging here was finished. As I lay in the upstairs bedroom that night, I could feel the gusts of the wind as they pummeled the house, hear the grating of heavy chains that held the floats to the shore, and feel the swell of the sea. A lonesome country, I thought, and yet I did not feel lonesome. I had friends.

It was still snowing the next day when Greg and I set out for his home in Nuchatlitz Inlet, near the Indian village of the same name. The rough sea pounded our small boat, and I was out of my seat more than I was in it.

"I hope you don't get seasick," Greg remarked dryly.

"I don't," I assured him.

"Good! We'll stop by your place on our way out. By the looks of things, this storm could keep up for a week. We may not get another chance."

Up Tahsis Inlet, through the narrow gap into Esperanza Inlet, past the mission hospital, then west down Esperanza Inlet to my cove, just a mile or so in from the open sea. After thirty miles of incessant pounding, I was ready for the stop.

There had been the same chill in the old house then, the same damp, musty odor that assailed me now, but a man's presence then spelled the difference. Coming in with Greg, it had not seemed too awful. The roof was leaking, a drop here, a drop there. We wiped up the floors and set buckets under the leaks. Now, my buckets were close to spilling over, and there was no one to help me.

I shook my head fiercely, as if by so doing I could dispel the past and face up to the present. Resolutely, I lifted the handle of the nearest bucket. The black bodies swished, sleek and shiny. I wanted to vomit, a momentary reflex I managed to stifle.

After a rainy season there was always an excess of water. Later I'd check the waterline, but at the moment it seemed best to get a fire going and get the chill out of the house. Such a wonderful stove! It had taken four men to carry the main section of the big kitchen range up to the cabin, but no electric stove could turn out cakes and pies of such perfection as came from my oven.

I patted it lovingly as I lifted the lids to lay my fire. The results were not what I'd expected. Smoke billowed from every seam in the old range and from between the stovepipe fittings. Tears streamed from my eyes as, coughing and choking, I ran for the door.

For the time being, that door would have to stay open. I'd always been careful to close every door, for hummingbirds will dart in through any opening and beat themselves to death against a windowpane in a frantic effort to escape. Certainly, I reasoned, no little hummingbird was likely to dart in through the billows of smoke now pouring out my door.

The fire would either smolder and die, or burn itself out. Now was as good a time as any to check the waterline. Swinging my bucket, I crossed over the first stream and followed the hose through the bushes along the shoreline. I found the break. Pressure from the winter rains had undoubtedly forced the hose apart. I tried to fix it, but my hands simply did not have the strength.

I filled my bucket in the pool dug by the first stream and climbed the bluff back to the house. The room still smelled of smoke, but I ventured in and looked up at my stovepipe, knowing this was where my trouble lay. A gentle tap on the pipe with a broom handle produced a dull thud. Loaded with soot, rusty, too, it would not stand much tapping. If I took the twelve-foot pipe apart, almost certainly I wouldn't be able to get it together again.

If I couldn't have a warm house, I would have a warm bed. I paused at the threshold of the living room. Sunlight pouring in through the west windows made this a pleasant room. It reflected softly against the pale apple green of the log walls and brightened the mahogany log beams across the ceiling. My eyes rested then upon the two upholstered rockers, one green, one pink, Wally's and mine, and I squeezed my eyes shut, as if by so doing I could blot out the memories.

When I opened them I found myself facing the small living-room heater. I was almost tempted. But those pipes were rusty, too, and no doubt full of soot. One smoldering fire in a day was enough. So I turned and climbed the stairs to the upstairs bedrooms. These rooms had always pleased me, bright and cheery when the sun came in. The ceilings sloped to two sides, and mahogany paneling from the floor to the slant of the ceiling gave the rooms added charm. I hummed to myself as I opened the storage chest and sorted out the bedding I would need. Then, my arms sagging from the weight, I made my way to the beach and spread it all—blankets, sheets, even the pillow—on the hot rocks.

It was a temptation to just sit there on those rocks and abandon my troubles, but more water had to be packed, and I was hungry, too. Minniebelle nodded approval as I lugged my buckets of water. The smoke had driven her away. I was glad she was back.

"You stick around, old girl," I said. "We'll make out."

And I was sure she answered, "Darn tootin' we will."

Food was not a pressing problem. There were a few tins stored in the pantry, and though the contents were not especially tempting cold, I could stomach it.

I decided to build a fire on the beach. Soon the fire was crackling and steam gushed from the teakettle spout. Pork and beans bubbled in a pot. I made my tea and I ate my beans from the pot, and nothing had ever tasted so good. I sat there by the fire, completely lost to the world, moving only to toss another stick on the flames. All thought processes had come to a standstill. But after a while I thought of my mother and a phrase she delighted in repeating.

"Trip lightly over trouble. It will not linger long."

So true! Plugged pipes and dead mice to the contrary, I was glad to be here. It was so quiet and peaceful. May evenings are long. The sun, reluctant to leave, casts a rosy glow, impregnating even the wee wisps of clouds. The rosy hues deepen, increasingly vivid. The sky, a miracle of changing colors, is reflected in the shimmering sea until sea meets sky in one glorious burst of crimson as the sun, in a final farewell, dips behind distant Mount Eliza.

I climbed the steps slowly, stopping to gaze back at a sky that still reflected the light of the sun.

Chapter 36

Oh, the beauty of sleep! Troubles evaporate. There's a quiet, an almost unearthly quiet. Unfortunately, the quiet did not last. It could have been any time past midnight when my sleep was disrupted by the persistent patter of little feet. Annoyed, I pulled the covers up around my ears, hoping to blot out the sound.

"Drat it, you kids!" I groped for my shoe beside the bed and slammed it against the wall. "Beat it! Go away!"

I did not have the courage to get up. In the ecstasy of their game the mice could easily patter over my feet. So I lay there, staring into the blackness, until the first streaks of a new day discouraged their frantic endeavors. I slept then, until the sun teased through my bedroom window. My bed was so cozy and warm, a striking contrast to the chill and dampness permeating the whole house, but the sun kept insisting, and I finally gave in. Oh, how I needed a cup of tea!

So it was back to the beach! With a fire going, a cup of hot tea in my hands, and a warm sun beating down on my back, the chill went out of my bones. Best of all, as I breathed in the sweet pure air, my spirits revived. I was ready to tackle the day. First I would walk around to the opposite side of the cove and inspect the little cottage Wally and I had purchased last summer, shortly before he died. Its purchase had made the entire cove our personal property. Oh, we'd felt rich—

two houses and 228 acres of land. I'd loved the cottage from the first, loved its quaint English style, its picturesque setting amid the trees. Yet yesterday, preoccupied with more pressing matters, I'd hardly given it a thought.

I approached the house slowly, paused at the threshold, admiring the floor-to-ceiling paneling, the ample bookshelves, and the circular corner cupboard.

I wandered into the kitchen, then the bedroom. Too bad there was a broken window and no stove. These three small rooms would be much easier to heat than the old log house. I wandered back outside, around to the back of the house and up the rock steps to the top of the bluff.

Out past the waters of my cove, beyond my diminutive islands, the choppy waters of the inlet were lined with evergreen mountains, and as far as I could see in any direction, there was no one but me. This did not depress me. There was, rather, a resurgence of the thrill I had felt when first we had come here.

But the day had certain demands. An old house waited to be swept and cleaned. Dishes and silver, pots and pans, all needed scalding, a tedious job under any circumstances, but when all the water must first be packed from a stream, then boiled over a fire on the beach, it is doubly difficult. Still, in my relaxed frame of mind, it did not seem insurmountable.

Dust was flying from the swish of my broom when a shout from the beach stopped me in my tracks.

"Who in the world?"

The shout came again, and with it, an inkling.

"Slim! Slim Beale!"

It had to be Slim. I'd written him from Seattle asking if he'd include me on his weekly run from Zeballos, at the head of Esperanza Inlet, to the fish camp at Queens Cove, where he delivered bread from the Zeballos bakery. Though Queens Cove was on the opposite side of the inlet and some little way up Port Eliza Inlet, I'd hoped Slim wouldn't object to the extra four or five miles to my place. Slim had written he'd come, but he hadn't said which day. Hope now put wings to my feet. I was barely conscious of the steps as I flew down them. He was sitting in a skiff, calm and unperturbed.

"Whoa! Whoa there! You'll break your neck tearing down those steps like that. I'll wait."

"Gosh, Slim! I'm so glad to see you."

"Figured you'd be. The pilot told me you'd gotten here. You didn't mention bringing anything in your letter, but I brought a couple loaves of bread anyway. Might go good."

"Sure will! Thanks, Slim. Where's your boat anyway?"

"Anchored on the far side of your islands. Can't get in here on a low tide, you know."

"I know! Well, next time I'll row out . . . if you'll help me get my skiff in the water."

"Sure thing," he said, edging up to the shore, then getting out and dragging his skiff up onto the rocks.

Slim was a strong man, very good-looking, blond with twinkling blue eyes and a smile that came easily. As he stood beside me I was conscious of my own slight five foot three inches and one hundred pounds.

He smiled. "Well, where have you got the boat hidden?"

"Back in the bushes. Mrs. McLean wrote that's where they put it after I left last September."

Slim eyed it with a decided skepticism. "Too heavy!" he said. "You can never manage this thing by yourself."

"Yes, I can," I insisted. "I'll keep it anchored out at about the half-tide mark."

"You can," Slim agreed, "but you'll get wet about every time you want to use it."

"So? I don't mind wading out, even swimming if I have to. I have plenty of rope. I can drop a light anchor from the stern, and with a long rope from the bow to this cedar here, I can haul it partway in when the tide's high. When the tide goes out I'll just keep shoving it out a little farther."

The blue eyes twinkled. "Sounds to me like you're going to be spending most of your time pulling or shoving. Well, okay! I guess you can do it. Let's get her in."

When the boat was in the water, Slim turned and said,

"Well, I'd best get moving. Anything you wanted next trip?"

"Oh, yes, there is! Stovepipes and mouse poison!"

"That's quite an order. Sounds like you might be having a mite of trouble."

"Sort of! The mice are awful, and the pipes are pretty badly rusted." I hesitated, biting my lower lip. "Maybe I shouldn't order them until I can find a man to put them up for me. Would you know anyone I could get?"

"Sure would! You're looking at him."

"Oh, Slim, I didn't mean it to be you."

"Don't be so picky," he retorted. "We're neighbors, aren't we? Even if we do live twenty miles apart! Any time a man can't lend a neighbor a hand! And by the way, are you planning to eat? So far your only concern has been to feed the mice."

His observation evoked a giggle. "I guess I do have to eat."

"Okay!" He pulled a note pad and pencil from his shirt pocket. "Write it down and I'll bring it next week."

I scribbled a few items, but as I handed the pad back to him, it was not food that was uppermost in my mind.

"You won't forget the pipes, Slim?"

Questioning eyes searched my face. "You sure you can get by for the week?"

"Oh, yes!" But I was careful not to mention that the pipes had deteriorated to a totally unusable state. Anyway, it was rather a lark having a fire on the beach, though Slim might not agree if he knew. In any event, I was firmly resolved to hold to that once-a-week service. If I weakened so soon, my summer could be just a series of concessions.

As I watched Slim row out, I realized I hadn't even mentioned that I'd never rowed a boat.

"Dumb!" I muttered to myself. "Well, this week I will learn."

That afternoon, in a burst of enthusiasm, I stoked up a real fire on my beach. It was lovely and warm, and the aroma of burning wood was pleasing. The effect was hypnotic. But the spell was broken when I spotted a speedboat approaching, and then another. Without realizing it, I had been sending up smoke signals. These were my Indian neighbors from Nuchatlitz, Rose and Alban Michael and a couple whose names I did not know. Rose and Alban had been our good friends ever since Wally and I had come to the island. I was glad to see them now.

"Picnic fire!" Rose exclaimed gleefully. "We see your smoke so we come in."

Everyone was in a gay mood, and since they expected a picnic, a picnic we would have. I made coffee on the grate over my flames, found a jar of peanut butter in the pantry, and, with the bread Slim had brought, made up some sandwiches.

We were sitting around the fire, laughing and joking, munching our sandwiches and sipping coffee, when Rose suddenly became serious.

"Alban is chief now," she said. "Felix say, 'I'm too old. I want Alban to be chief!'"

"Alban!" I exclaimed. "That's wonderful."

"Yes," Alban agreed. "But my father is wise. He has much to say yet."

I nodded. "That's good."

The other Indian woman spoke up—Tillie, they called her. "Yes, it is good. Now Alban is our king and Rose is our queen. We do what they say."

Rose giggled shyly, and Alban smiled, nodding his head. It was evident they were both pleased.

Suddenly I remembered to tell them about my waterline.

"Do you think you could fix it, Alban?" I asked.

He nodded. "We see!"

Strong hands were all that was needed. Alban was pleased to have helped me, and now I would have water in my kitchen.

We strolled back to the fire. My Indian friends were in no hurry to leave, and I was glad to have them stay, but after a while I began to wonder if I really did have water in my kitchen. Excusing myself, I ran up the steps, opened the door, then stopped in dismay. I did have water in the kitchen—in fact, all over the kitchen. The hose leading into the sink had sprunk a leak, a big leak. The hose would have to be replaced. I ran outside to shut off the valve, then back down the steps to tell my friends. The mess I would clean up later.

My announcement was greeted with bursts of laughter. Mrs. Flynn had water. She had water all over the house. It was a big joke. It began to seem funny even to me, and I joined in the laughter. My friends went away happy, leaving me to cope with my problem. Somehow, up here it was just another occurrence, one that had to be taken in stride.

Chapter 37

That night I was awakened by rain on the roof. The elements had conspired against me. I shivered in my bed, dreading the day.

As I forced myself out of bed, my determination to enjoy cold food soon faltered. It was no lark now to have a fire on the beach. Just keeping it going tested my ingenuity as it sputtered its protest against the rain.

I counted the days until Slim would be back, and I wondered if I could ever hold out.

I rebuked myself. "Of course you'll hold out. What else can you do? You can't phone Zeballos and say, 'Come and get me.' You haven't a phone." I paused for a giggle that was partly chagrin. "Come to think of it, they haven't a phone, either."

But the giggle made me feel better, and the first wisps of steam were rising from my teakettle spout. I knelt on the rocks and made my tea. The world I surveyed now was vastly different from the bright world that had entranced me, was it only yesterday? My mountains had vanished as if a curtain had been drawn. The birds had all sought the deep brush. Even Minniebelle had not been out to greet me. I felt deserted.

When I returned to the house I found it colder inside than out, and the sight of the pots and pans I'd set out to catch the drips from my shingled roof did nothing to heighten my spirits.

Glumly, I wandered into the living room. My eyes strayed to the small wood heater, and I could not pull them away. A forlorn hope tugged at my muddled brain. True, the pipes were loose and rusty, but if I maneuvered them ever so gently, maybe I could slip them into place. I was careful, and they did slip into place, but when I took my hands away I was left staring at a hole the size of both hands.

I remembered those small sheets of aluminum I'd seen in the woodshed. The tin snips were dull, and I tried fruitlessly to cut the aluminum until my hands ached. Bending it was no easier, but I persisted, finally putting it between my knees, using them to exert the pressure my hands could not. That worked, and I was proud of my accomplishment until it occurred to me that I'd have to hold the aluminum in place.

I chewed at my lip, a bad habit, but a help, as I concentrated on this new problem. There had to be a way. "I bet there's a roll of bandaging tape in Wally's bag."

I rummaged in Wally's bag and found the tape. Fingers trembling, I applied it across the aluminum and around the pipe, fearful I'd puncture yet another hole. But the pipe didn't give way, and the patch held. Hallelujah! I risked a very small fire, but when I stood close, huddling near the stove, I could feel a faint warmth. It was good.

It continued to rain, and I kept counting the days. My world had become noisy, my streams cascading in boisterous abandon over their rocky beds. I still cooked my meals on the beach, for the occasional small fire I chanced in my heater gave off barely enough heat to warm my hands. And every day I bailed out my skiff and, ignoring the rain trickling down my neck, attempted to row. Never would I have believed a boat could be so contrary. Against my every effort, it seemed determined to go in circles. And as I struggled I thought of my friends in Seattle, snug in their luxurious homes, every convenience at their fingertips.

"What do you do up there all day?" more than one had asked, as if, really, there were nothing to do at all. Would they ever believe it took every minute of the day just to stay alive?

And all the time I kept counting the days. Four more to go. Three. Two. At last, the day! I'd been on the beach for hours, straining to see through the rain and the mist, listening for the first faint whine of an engine. I heard it long before I saw it, waiting, before climbing into my skiff, to make certain it was Slim's boat. My rowing was still erratic, my course far from straight. Slim had already anchored his water taxi and was waiting for me to pull alongside. A grin spread over his face, but his words were encouraging.

"You're doing okay," he said.

I gave him an answering grin, knowing full well my best was not good. I was quivering with excitement. New stovepipes at last! Nothing else mattered. He handed down a box of groceries and then a packet of mail, but he didn't say a word about the pipes, just stood there in the rain smiling down at me, as if our business were finished. Could he possibly have forgotten? Fighting a troubling uncertainty, I mustered the courage to ask.

"No, I didn't forget," he assured me with a smile. "Witton's store was out of your size, though, so I had to order them. They should be in on the *Uchuck* in a couple of days."

"Gosh!" I said, feigning unconcern, hoping no quaver betrayed me. "I've sorta been counting the days. A fire on the beach doesn't work too well in the rain."

A look of consternation replaced the grin. "You mean you haven't had a fire in that old range all this time?"

I nodded, not trusting myself to speak. Disappointment had brought such a lump in my throat that I couldn't even swallow over it.

"Can you make out until Thursday?" he asked.

I nodded again. Thursday was but two days away. And then I found my voice.

"It's not all that bad, really."

Thoughtful eyes searched my face, took in my wet clothes. I met the look, my own eyes unwavering. We both knew I had lied. We both also knew I would stick it out, because I could have asked him to take me to town, if necessary.

Slim left, and it rained harder than ever. I sat huddled by the tiny fire in my heater, listening to the beat of the rain on the roof, to the ping of each raindrop as it found its way in, playing musical tunes in my pots and pans.

Thursday came and it was still raining. I was in a fever of uncertainty. Would Slim come in the rain to put up my pipes? In my heart I was sure he would. Another disappointment would be too hard to bear. I stayed away from the beach, determined to be dispassionate, but my ears were primed for that first whine of an engine.

It came at last, faintly at first. I stood in the doorway, my head cocked to one side. Each engine has its own individual intonation. Yes! It was Slim's boat. I was down the steps and into my skiff so fast I wasn't quite sure how I got there.

Slim shook his head when he saw me. "You ought to put some clothes on. You're wet to the skin. You'll catch your death."

"No I won't," I retorted, pushing wet hair away from my eyes. "I've been out every day and I've not even a sniffle. I guess shorts don't look too practical, but they're practical for me when I have to wade out to the skiff. I can't stand wet pants flapping around my legs."

"Maybe not, but it sure wouldn't hurt to wear a jacket and something on your head."

"I know! I forgot!"

His eyes twinkled. "You really want those pipes, don't you? Okay, here you are . . . one at a time so you don't drop one overboard. Now, how about you sitting in the stern? I'll row us in. I'm a mite heavier than you, I figure."

He could also set a course and stay on it, though he didn't say so. I was happy to let him row.

Slim eyed my pipes dubiously when we got to the house, and I held my breath. Would he still want to tackle the job?

"Darn things are liable to fall apart when I take them down," he said. "If you've got some old newspapers, you'd better spread them around. We're going to have one hell of a mess."

"It's okay. I can clean it up."

"Spread out the papers anyway. They'll catch some of it. Now, if this old stove will hold me, I think I can work best from there."

"It'll hold you. Wally used to stand on it."

As Slim worked, soot and bits of rusted pipe floated about the room. Soot was everywhere, infiltrating the air. My lungs protested and I coughed, but there was not a word of complaint from Slim. He even smiled as he handed down the first section of pipe. I carried it outside, then another and another. The worst was over, I figured, but putting up those new pipes wasn't as simple a job as I'd anticipated. The pipe lengths had to fit snugly so no smoke could escape. The length that fitted onto the stove had to be bent and shaped.

"Well," Slim observed as he jumped down from the top of the stove, "that ought to hold you for a while. What about this stove now? Have you cleaned it out?"

"No," I admitted, "but I will. I know how."

"I'll give you a hand. Want to make darn sure this stove's functioning before I take off."

Slim made a fire after he'd finished. There was a soft crackling as the kindling caught, and no smoke!

"I can't ever thank you enough, Slim."

"You have," he said, and he was grinning. "You should see yourself. You're black as this stove, but I've never seen a happier face."

A quick look in the mirror confirmed his observation. I was black, all right, face and arms, but my eyes were shining. Already my kitchen had begun to feel warm. I'd fill my teakettle and some big pans and soon I'd have hot water. With soap and hot water I could accomplish miracles.

"Could you stay for coffee, Slim?" I asked.

"No, sorry! Some other time. That old boat of mine sort of pokes along. It'll be late now before I get home."

I walked with him down to the beach. Water was boiling when I got back to the house. I was tempted to sit down for that hot cup of tea, but I could see the mess now and I couldn't ignore it. I gathered up papers. I swept. I dusted. Finally, I scrubbed myself. I felt cozy, relaxed, almost smug.

I set my tea on the table, found paper and a pen, and pulled up a chair. Then I started to write, letters to Maureen, to Mama, to my sister, Berne. The chill and the ache had gone out of my hands. It was good to be able to hold a pen. Intent on my writing, a faint sizzling and sputtering somewhere behind me made little impression. The sizzle became more persistent. It puzzled me vaguely, but still I ignored it. At last, annoyed, I glanced over my shoulder, then leaped from my chair. The pan under the pipe that extended through the roof was catching not only stray raindrops but red-hot coals. Peering up into the jacket around the pipe, I could see it was filled with those burning coals.

"Oh, no!" And I scratched my head as I puzzled over this newest predicament. That pipe and the jacket had looked to be in good condition. Slim had not replaced it. Evidently, though, it contained bits of tar and pitch which had been dislodged when Slim inserted the connecting pipe. The roaring fire in the stove, which had so pleased me, had heated the pipe and ignited the pitch.

"It'll burn out eventually, I suppose," I said to myself, "but darn, it might burn my pipe out, too. I could climb up on the roof and pour water down the pipe." I frowned, debating the results.

Pulling my chair over to the pipe, I climbed up on it, glaring up at the burning coals. Around the bottom of the jacket were small holes, about the circumference of a pen. If there was just some way I could get those coals out. And then I had an inspiration. With a screwdriver I could poke into those holes and work the coals out.

How long I worked, my head tipped back, my arms stretched over my head, I don't know, but the kink in my neck and the ache in my arms attested that it was too long. When I jumped down from the chair, my fingers were cramped and I'd lost any urge to write.

Chapter 38

The days passed and it didn't rain anymore. I cut brush, freeing my windows. Though Wally and I had cleared it before, brush fills in quickly. Pricked fingers, scratched arms, and aching muscles are powerful dissuaders, but my determination increased with the increase of light within my kitchen.

Minniebelle wasn't in complete accord with my ambitious endeavors. The brush was her haunt. In its impenetrable tangle she laid her eggs and brought forth her young. Wally and I had seen it happen, as she fed her family on the salmonberries and the thimbleberries which turned a bright red in July and on the salalberries which had taken on a rich purple hue. Now she perched far back in the brush, eyeing me dourly, or stomped across the kitchen roof, each stomp an expression of disapproval.

She also disapproved of my efforts to chop wood. The thud of the ax, the ring of metal against metal as sledgehammer met wedge, set off an angry flutter of wings as Minniebelle took off for a quieter and safer perch. She didn't trust my aim any more than I did. As the slabs fell apart, the chunks flew. My arms and legs were covered with bruises. I soon learned to jump very fast. Swing the sledgehammer and jump back. Swing again and jump back. It didn't work too well, however, as Slim's observation attested the next time he came in.

"What in God's name are you doing to yourself?"

"Nothing. I was just chopping wood is all."

"Chopping wood! If anyone happened in here and got a look at you, they'd think for sure I'd attacked you."

"Probably no one will come in. Anyway, I have to chop wood. My stove eats it up."

"Okay! You have to chop wood, but let me show you how. You're probably trying to pound your way through every blasted knot."

It was true, I admitted silently. I had let the ax fall where it would, it never having occurred to me it would be easier and simpler to cut on either side of a knot. If the ax stuck, I'd pound it on through with the sledgehammer. I hadn't really been chopping wood. I'd been massacring it. Even now my ax was embedded. The whine of Slim's engine had stayed my efforts to free it. He shook his head when he saw.

"It's a wonder either you or the ax survived."

I wondered what people, away off somewhere, were doing, but I had a world of my own. The squirrels chattered at me. The discordant call of the blue jay was music to my ears and the flash of blue wings in flight a delight to the eye. From my perch on the beach I watched my favorite mink swim out for a fish. He shook the fish vigorously, making sure of his kill, then trotted for the bush, ignoring me completely, though his path led almost over my feet.

I waited, sometimes hours, for Oscar, the seal, to come in. Friendly and curious, he considered my harbor his private domain. What a showoff he was, swimming swiftly underwater, popping up, always facing me, as if demanding, "Well, how was that?" Sometimes I was sure he said, "Come and play." My swimming prowess, matched against his, could be nothing but ludicrous.

No creature feared me, not the mink or the seal or the hummingbirds that darted past my ear. I didn't mind their mischievous swoops so long as they didn't shove that stiletto beak in for a test. The sea gulls and the crows ignored me. I was part of the world that was theirs and I belonged. And always there was Minniebelle to back me up.

I learned many lessons. I learned to run over the rocks, as sure-footed as a mountain goat, spotting in advance those rocks which could shift and throw me off balance. I learned never to be startled, not even when a snake would slither across my path, or even the day when a scraping and clawing on my roof suggested some sizable animal had failed to gain footing.

There were cougar about. That clawing sound on my roof was not made by a squirrel. A cat is sure-footed, but the pitch of my roof was steep. A cat leaping from a nearby cedar could find his footing insecure.

My feelings, as I ran outside, were of curiosity, not fear. If that was a cougar that had landed on my roof, I wanted to see it. I circled the house. Nothing. I climbed a ladder. The claw marks on my roof were indecisive.

"I'll never know. And I won't dare tell anyone. They'll only think my imagination is working overtime."

One day, however, someone did come—a face appeared at my window. I was surprised. It was not a face I knew. And I hadn't heard a boat, which was strange, for my ears were attuned to the sounds of a boat. The faintest chug or whine would send me racing to the beach. Was it the Indians going in to Zeballos for supplies or to the hospital at Esperanza? Often it was a troller. Most all the Indian families had trollers. White fishermen, too, were coming into the area.

Now I was puzzled. That face at my window belonged to a young man, a white man. Still wondering who he could be and how he had arrived, I pushed back from the table and went to the door.

"Hello."

"Hello," he replied.

We stood staring at each other.

"I didn't expect to find anyone living here," he said finally.

"You know this place then?"

"No. I'm new in this area. I work at the mill in Tahsis. Left my boat at the river about a quarter of a mile from here. Decided to hike along the shore . . . just happened on your house."

"Well, that solves my mystery. Couldn't understand why I didn't hear a boat." I looked at him speculatively. He seemed a nice enough young man. "Would you care for a cup of coffee?"

"Sure would! Never dreamt the shoreline was so rugged. It's quite a hike around those cliffs. Almost turned back a couple of times."

He came in and sat down, and I made coffee. It was pleasant, for a change, to have someone besides Minniebelle to talk to. I sat relaxed, one leg crossed over the other, unconsciously swinging a foot. Of a sudden a little mouse darted between me and my guest. A startled look on his face was replaced by one of incredulity. I made no comment. My foot was still swinging.

"Didn't you . . . didn't you see that mouse?" His voice, too, was incredulous. I could read his thoughts. Women didn't just sit with mice playing about.

I'd learned to tolerate them, at least to a degree. I smiled when I spoke, quite composed. "Yes, I saw him. They do run around a bit."

His excuse for leaving was incoherent. He almost ran from my door, and as he disappeared I wondered, Was it me or was it the mouse?

Chapter 39

Early one hot afternoon a little boat came puttering along right up to my beach. While they were still at a distance I had identified the passengers as Indians. No white man would have ventured out in such a frail craft. There were four in the boat, a man and a woman and two small children.

They made their approach in silence. Not even a hand was raised in greeting. Although I didn't know their names, I recalled having seen them at Nuchatlitz. Baffled, but not wanting to appear unfriendly, I called out a cheery hello. There was no response. Then the engine was silenced, and, tentatively, I tried again.

"Hello?" In that one word I hoped to convey my hospitality, but it came out more as a question.

The man climbed from his boat, dragged it partway up on the rocks, then lifted the children out and sat them on the rocks. The word he used was not familiar to me, but the children, like puppets on a string, folded themselves onto the rocks. The woman remained in the boat, eyes focused straight ahead, seeming to see neither me nor the children.

My concern turned to consternation when the man shoved the boat from the rocks and, for the first time, turned to face me.

"You take care," he said. "We come back."

In one motion, it seemed, he was in the boat and had the

engine running. Without even a backward glance, they chugged out through the channel and into the inlet. Their departure brought howls of dismay from the children, though they remained as if glued to the spot where they'd been commanded to sit. My dismay matched theirs, if indeed it did not exceed it. The parents—certainly they must be the parents—had given no clue to where they were going or when they might return. They were headed toward Zeballos, but they could be going into Tahsis Inlet and on down to Friendly Cove. They could be gone days.

This was no wild supposition. I knew Indian children were often left at the mission hospital at Esperanza while the parents went off on some unexplained errand. The children were always sick, the parents insisted, a bad cold if nothing else. Maybe I'd been elected to baby-sit instead of the nurses.

Both children were screaming at the top of their lungs; the sounds reverberated across the cove and into the hills. For the first time since my arrival at the cove, I felt fear. But then my heart went out to them, poor little waifs, sitting so forlornly on the rocks, wiping their tearstained faces with dirty fists. There must be something I could do.

Food. Of course! Even the most unhappy child would find it hard to ignore a treat. I ran up the steps to the house, ignoring as well as I could their cries, which seemed to increase in volume. The children must have thought I was deserting them, too. Rummaging through my cupboards, I came upon a bag of peanuts, a gift from Slim on one of his visits.

I raced back to the beach, popped a peanut into each mouth. Though their big, round brown eyes were full of distrust, the crying subsided. They accepted more peanuts, evidently having decided I wasn't too monstrous, and I began to wonder what I had here . . . boys, girls? Their black hair was cropped short and they were both dressed alike, in jeans. I judged their ages to be about four and five. I tried to question them, but the round, unblinking brown eyes were uncomprehending. English, it seemed, wasn't one of their accomplishments. No matter. There were other ways to make myself understood.

I wondered, then, were they housebroken? There was one way to find out. I took a child by each hand and led them up to my outhouse. Speaking slowly and very distinctly, I said, "Now, every time, you come here."

And so they did, taking me by the hand, an insistent tug demanding I go with them. At least one mystery was solved. I had a boy and a girl.

My suspicion that I had replaced the nurses at the hospital was soon confirmed. In my shorts and shirt I bore slight resemblance to a nurse, but to these children it made no difference. I was Nurse. And in that one word I took some small comfort. It was communication of a sort. With this assurance, I dared more questions, and they answered with a nod or a negative shake of the head. It gave me a feeling of authority and with it a realization that, whether or not they spoke English, they understood it to a degree. There was, however, no exchange of words between the two, no attempt at play. Except for the trips up to the outhouse, they just sat there on the rocks, staring at me, their brown eyes serious and unwavering. How did one entertain such guests? I had nothing a child could play with. It had been years since I'd had any practice inventing games. Maybe a nap. After all, they were very young.

I went up to the house for blankets, then chose a grassy spot under a mountain ash and fixed up a bed. Wondering brown eyes watched my every movement. When I summoned them to come and lie down, they obeyed unquestioningly. I covered them over, patted their heads, hoping the pats would give them a measure of assurance.

"Go to sleep," I said, and I sat down to watch them.

The small bodies never moved. They lay as if staked to that tree, but the eyes never closed. Obviously they didn't want to sleep. I had been thinking only of myself.

"Okay," I said. "Time to get up." And I pulled back the blanket.

What a strange person they must think me, but as they sat up I was rewarded with a shy smile from the girl, and I felt good. Nurse or whatever, I'd been accepted.

"Water," she said.

Ah! Another word! But of course they were thirsty—all those peanuts. So I got two cups from the kitchen, then led them to the stream and pointed out the pool where I dipped. They drank and they drank. The water in the stream, shaded by towering evergreens and thick underbrush, was cool and refreshing. So good! I could see it in the exchanged glances, in the light that had finally appeared in the somber brown eyes.

A tug on my hand meant another trip to the outhouse. It became a game—down to the stream for water, up the steps of the embankment to the outhouse to expel it. I was sure the need for the frequency of those trips was greatly exaggerated, but it was something to do. Much better than sitting on the rocks! It was fun, the eyes said, and Nurse could share in the fun. Indeed, Nurse was forced to play the game. The moist grip of those little hands in mine granted no reprieve. And all the time I kept watching, hoping. Surely the parents would come back.

My hope waned with the lowering progress of the sun in the western sky. Suppertime and still no sign of a boat. And I was tired. But the children must be fed. I debated. I could take them up to the house, but I hadn't had a fire in the stove all day. It would be just as easy to have a fire on the beach, and on the beach I could watch. There was still plenty of reflected light in that western sky. The parents could still return.

I looked at my charges. Though they had paddled their hands in the water on every trip to the stream, they were still in need of a good scrubbing. This time I led the way—up to the kitchen. I got soap, filled a basin with water, and rolled up the sleeves of their knit tops. Astonishment halted the proceedings. Exposed on bare arms were their names, painstakingly lettered in black ink.

"Larry?" I asked. "Lorraine?"

Vigorous nods answered my questions. Smiles brightened their faces. No longer were they nameless. Impulsively, I pulled them to me and hugged them tight. They were such good children, not at all disobedient.

"Okay," I said, "let's get washed up. Then you can help me with supper."

With children, it seems, an activity either is fun or it isn't. Supper on the beach was fun. Larry and Lorraine ran to gather firewood, almost tripping over each other in their eagerness, seeming to spot the same piece of wood at the same time. They took turns, running back and forth, their arms sagging from the weight of the wood. I could almost forget I had hoped their parents would soon come back.

After supper my worry returned. I boiled water and washed the dishes, and all the while I looked out to sea, but no little boat reappeared. Nearly nine o'clock. The children should be in bed, even though there was still light in the sky, even though their parents might still come. Maybe the davenport would serve. Old-fashioned and overly generous, it had room and to spare for two small bodies. So I made up a bed there and tucked them in, one at each end.

"Larry! Lorraine! Go to sleep now."

And they did.

I went back to the beach, dismayed at the sight of a heavy black cloud building up over Mount Eliza. Then a sudden brisk wind churned the seas. I watched and I fretted. Their boat was too small. I glanced at my watch . . . a quarter past ten. The sea was running strong now, with a heavy chop, and the night sky was far from reassuring. It was foolish to stay longer on the beach.

With one last backward glance, I climbed the steps to my house, and I sighed a little sigh of relief. I lit my lamp and went into the living room to check on my charges. I had to smile. Wanted or unwanted, how peaceful they were in sleep. I went back to the kitchen, sat down at the table.

Then I heard voices. Impossible! I cocked my head to the

side, holding my breath as I listened. Grabbing up a flashlight, I ran for the beach. There were the parents, dragging their boat up over the rocks.

"What happened?" I demanded. "It's so late. I've been worried."

"Engine broke down," the father explained. "We row but can get nowhere. Sea too rough."

It seemed silly to waste time asking further questions, but I had to know.

"If you couldn't row against the sea, how did you get here?"

"Troller take us in tow. We take the kids now and go home."

"But you can't," I protested. "They're asleep. Besides, I don't see the troller."

"It waits on the other side of your islands. Too many reefs here."

The night was too stormy, the sea kicking up too much of a fuss, but Larry and Lorraine were their children. There was no way I could stop them. I watched helplessly as the children were snatched from their bed, carried whimpering down to the boat, and told to be quiet. They looked up at me, eyes imploring, and I ached to snatch them up in my arms.

Already the boat had shoved off. I watched, unmoving, as the father strained at the oars, the waves curling and breaking. It would be a long hard pull to the far side of my islands. Could he make it? Then the night swallowed them up, and all I could see was the wicked curl of the sea as it lashed the shore at my feet. Though I'd had those children but one day, their innocence, the utter simplicity with which they had accepted me, had worked a small miracle. What happened to them now mattered . . . oh, so much. With a heavy heart I turned again to the steps.

Worried, preoccupied, I was slowly preparing for bed when some instinct directed my attention to the door. There was a face at the windows. The Indian father! How long had he been there? I hadn't heard a sound. Hastily rebuttoning my shirt, I went to the door.

"The boat go away." He stated it simply, without anger.

The story came out slowly. They had rowed out around the islands, buffeted by the wind and the sea, only to find the troller had deserted them. Perhaps it had been unable to hold anchor. There was nothing then the Indian family could do but row back to my shores.

"But where is your wife, your children?" I asked as he finished his recital.

"They wait in the boat."

Of course! They waited for the invitation. "Bring them up," I said.

The childen went back on the davenport, and I made up a bed upstairs for the parents. I asked their names. Matthew and Margaret, they said. Then the conversation stopped. I could think of nothing to say, and they seemed content to just sit and say nothing. It was past eleven o'clock, and I was tired. Why didn't they go on up to bed?

At last Matthew was moved to speech. "I've been on a kind of a diet today," he said.

"You have?" I asked the obvious question, but more out of politeness than interest.

"Yes," he volunteered. "I haven't eaten all day."

My mouth dropped open, but no words came. At this late hour food had been the furthest thing from my mind, but I built a fire and cooked their supper, and when finally I fell into bed, I didn't even wonder if they were comfortable. I just went to sleep.

The next morning, quite early, I heard footsteps, but I was sleepy and chose to ignore them. Some while later I heard those footsteps coming up the stairs. They stopped at my bedroom door. The door had swelled during the damp winter months, so that I'd not been able to close it properly. Through the open door, Matthew informed me he'd been up for hours. He'd been working on his engine and had it repaired.

"We eat and then we go," he finished.

I got up. There was no alternative. I made a big breakfast, and when my guests were satisfied, I walked with them down to the beach. The sea was calm now, unrippled, belying the night's storm. Matthew's lips parted in a smile.

"She's a good engine," he said. "I am happy she is fixed. I would not want my wife to have to row home. Such a long way! It is too hard for her."

Margaret made no comment. Indeed, she had hardly uttered a word their entire stay. I waved to the children and watched until the boat was out of sight, also glad that Margaret didn't have to row home.

I had thought the incident was over, but some days later, when I was out prowling my beach, I spotted a speedboat approaching. It was well throttled back, barely moving. It stopped, started again, veering from side to side. Was it in trouble? No, it was still moving. But what was that rolling behind? Could it be? Yes, it was. That boat was towing a log and it was coming into my cove. As it came closer I recognized a young friend from Nuchatlitz.

"Pat!" I called. "I haven't seen you in a long time."

He grinned, but he didn't return my greeting. He was busy. He didn't want his boat to scrape on my rocks, so he dropped his anchor offshore. Then he waded to shore, a power saw gripped under his arm. Pat is taller than most of his people. His shoulders were broad, and he carried the saw easily. His eyes were smiling as he came up beside me, but his voice was solemn.

"When the tide goes out I will cut you some wood."

That it would be several hours before the tide went out far enough to allow that log to sit on the rocks concerned Pat not at all. My neighbors at Nuchatlitz, I had learned through the years, were untroubled by urgency. There was always time. Pat waded back out to the boat and returned carrying a small salmon.

"I just happened to catch it on the way over," he explained.

I realized suddenly that I was being repaid for my hospitality to Matthew and Margaret. I realized also that a service to any one of them was a service to all, that the one you helped wouldn't necessarily be the one who repaid you. What these people do is done simply, matter-of-factly. I didn't embarrass Pat now with any great outpouring of thanks. Instead I said, "Could I fix you some dinner while we wait for the tide to go out?"

If I had put this question to a white person he would probably have said, "Well, it would be nice, if it won't put you to too much trouble."

But Indian people do not waste a lot of words. Pat said, "Yes," and followed me up to the house.

I tried to make conversation, but it was mostly questions on my part and a simple yes or no on his. But his eyes were friendly, and he was completely relaxed as he drank cup after cup of coffee, well diluted with canned milk and sweetened with several teaspoons of sugar.

I felt compelled to keep speaking even though Pat gave no answers. He kept smiling in a tolerant manner until finally he decided it was time to check the log. It was good to have such friends, and to Pat, in particular, I was especially grateful, for when he left there was much wood stacked in my woodshed and a beautiful salmon waiting to be baked.

Chapter 40

It was the middle of July, and my mother was coming to visit me. I had agreed to her visit against my better judgment. A woman seventy-four years old shouldn't be running around on my rocky beach, with no communication and Slim a week away. However, my mother is very persuasive, also very determined. She wanted to see where I lived, and see it she would.

Since I couldn't deter her, I decided to have a man come at the same time to do some much needed work around the place. Discounting the work, I'd be happy to have him around. I put my fears aside to revel in the anticipation of her visit.

The day arrived, sunny and warm, and the cove more enchanting than any South Sea island paradise. In a little while Slim would be bringing Mama out, and probably Mr. Allard, too, to fix up my house. I scurried about getting things ready, making the beds, sweeping my floors clean of the evergreen needles I was forever tracking in. In the midst of all this bustle there came a shrill whistle. I'd heard the drone of an engine from my kitchen, had felt the vibration, but chalked it off as a passing freighter. Now I paused in my work, frowning. Ordinarily the blare of a whistle would have sent me racing to the beach. Today, I didn't welcome the interruption. It couldn't be Slim. Another blare, more demanding, shattered the silence of my kitchen.

"Oh, darn!" I muttered as I raced for the beach. There I stopped in my tracks. Sitting off my islands was the *Uchuck*, the freight and passenger boat that made runs from Gold River to Zeballos. I could see people lining the deck, could hear their voices, their laughter, and I knew where the *Uchuck* was heading. The mission at Esperanza had a summer Bible camp at Ferrier Point, a twenty-mile run from the mission, out past Nuchatlitz, out in the Pacific to a peninsular point of land that formed a breakwater for the camp. It would have been difficult to get all their camp equipment out there in their small boats, so they had chartered the *Uchuck*. The gestures were clear—they wanted me to row out and come along.

I cupped my hands and I shouted, "I can't come." But the wind was from the wrong direction, and the words rang mockingly in my ears as they faded into nothingness. I waved and motioned them to go away.

Their answer was another blast from the whistle. I'd have to row out and tell them I couldn't go. I'd practiced rowing faithfully, but the short hauls to meet Slim, always within the confines of my islands, was child's play in comparison to what was expected of me now. My heart beat like a tom-tom within the walls of my chest. My fingertips tingled as I rubbed them together.

A double toot, more insistent, sent me out to my skiff. Whatever, I had to go.

The sea wasn't too choppy, I discovered when I got out there. My misgivings had magnified their gentle rise and fall into something portentous. I pulled hard on the oars, pride in each stroke. I could see the people plainly now. Their voices encouraged me. One voice rang out above the others, clear as a bell.

"Bethine!"

I glanced up, startled, disbelieving. Mama? It couldn't be. But it was. Whatever was she doing on this ship? There was no time to puzzle it out. Already my skiff had nudged the side, a rope ladder had been lowered, and one of the crew was descending. Captain George McCandless was leaning over the railing, grinning down at me.

"Come on up," he said. "We're taking this bunch out to Ferrier. You can come along for the ride."

A sling was lowered, two heavy canvas straps. The crewman positioned them on my skiff fore and aft. I caught the ladder as it swung by me and scrambled up the side of the ship, reaching up for Captain George's outstretched hand. He pulled me aboard, but there was no time for talk. My skiff, with the crewman clinging to the straps, was out of the water, swinging free in the air. People pushed back out of the way as the hoist lifted it up and over the railing, depositing it gently on the deck of the *Uchuck*. People pushed forward then, calling out my name. Somehow I made my way to Mama.

"I don't know what this is all about," she said as she hugged me, "but I've never had such fun. Do you know where we're going?"

"I do," and I explained about the summer Bible camp.

"And we get to go along for the ride! Isn't that nice!" She rattled on, almost in the same breath, "The captain of this boat is the nicest man. When he found out I was your mother, do you know what he said?"

I made no attempt to conceal my amusement. "I can guess, but tell me anyway."

"Well, he said, 'No mother of Bethine's is going to walk up that long dusty road in Zeballos to go to a hotel.' Then he got a bit of a twinkle in his eye and he said, 'That hotel's kind of a rough place. Bethine wouldn't forgive us if we let you get in trouble. We'll keep you here with us, where we can keep an eye on you.'"

I laughed outright. "Sounds like George, all right."

She wasn't finished. "The meals I had! Steak for supper last night, bacon and eggs for breakfast this morning, and all the cocoa I could drink. They fixed a bed for me last night. Put the table down somehow so it was even with the benches and curtained it all off. I've never felt so special."

"You are special." George was beside us, an arm around

each of us. "The cook has lunch ready. Better come and join us."

Mama took the trip in stride, the roll of the boat in the ocean swells, the clamor of the youngsters, the excitement of unloading at Ferrier as stoves, mattresses, even a jeep were hoisted over the side and onto a small barge, which would be towed in as far as possible, then allowed to sit until the outgoing tide left it exposed on the sand. Three hours later we approached my cove. Mama's enthusiasm hadn't dimmed.

"To think I had to wait all these years for a trip like this," she exulted.

A brisk wind had sprung up, kicking up the sea, and the tide was on its way out. The *Uchuck* had to anchor far out from my islands. Pitting my strength against the wind and the tide, especially with Mama's added weight, would be a real test. Mama was not much taller than I, but she was heavier. But my skiff, with a crewman aboard, had been lowered back into the sea. The ladder was dropped down, and I went over the side. The crewman held the ladder snug as Mama descended. She showed no fear of the ladder, calmly descending, the blackness of her coat standing out against the whiteness of the ship. I wondered briefly if she could know what courage she had, entrusting herself to my bobbing little boat with me at the oars.

She was down and seated in the stern. Once Mama and I were alone in a boat I wasn't sure I could handle, I took an oar and pushed hard against the hull of the ship to give us some leeway. It was a start. I pulled hard on both oars, for a few minutes making some headway, the *Uchuck* a bulwark against the force of the wind. But out beyond the protection it offered, I found myself floundering. I braced my feet against the floorboards and strained at the oars with all the strength I could muster, but the distance between my boat and the islands did not lessen. Could I make it? I knew the crew of the *Uchuck* were watching and wondering, too. And Mama? Was she frightened? I looked back at her. She was holding on with both hands, but her smile was serene. She actually believed I could do it. I pulled hard at the oars, and it did seem the distance was lessening . . . maybe. Then suddenly, from out of nowhere, a speedboat pulled up beside me, and I recognized Vera, Pat's wife.

"You want a tow?" she called out.

Gratefully, I nodded my head, too tired for speech. I tossed her a line, then turned to wave to the crew of the *Uchuck*. Their engine throbbed in answer and they were on their way.

Vera helped me get Mama ashore without wetting her feet. We put a plank from the prow to the shore and steadied Mama as she walked it. Then we all went up to the house and had coffee.

Vera, like Pat, was not much inclined to conversation. I wondered how Mama would make out with her. I needn't have worried. Mama didn't ask a lot of questions that required a yes or no answer. She didn't ask any questions at all. Mama liked to tell jokes. She told every joke she knew and each time Vera rewarded her with peals of laughter. Oh, Mama was enjoying those jokes, too. Her blue eyes twinkled as she laughed along with Vera. She told the joke about the young lover who walked his sweetheart by a popcorn wagon.

"My, that popcorn smells good!" the young girl exclaimed.

"It does," her lover agreed. "Shall we walk back by and smell it again?"

I wasn't sure Vera had ever smelled popcorn. I was certain a popcorn wagon was quite beyond anything she would have experienced. Yet she liked the joke.

When Mama and I were alone, the lecture began. I told her all the things she must not do because she was in her seventies and I didn't want her to get hurt. Don't go down the steps to the beach by yourself. Don't wander alone too far in the woods. Above all, don't try to cut kindling. Mama gave me a bright little smile, but not a word did she say. I knew she'd bear watching.

Later that afternoon Slim came in, bringing Mr. Allard. "I didn't even get a peek at your mother," Slim protested. "George kidnapped her."

"I know," I replied, laughing. "But you'll be taking both

her and Mr. Allard out in a couple of weeks. You'll get to know her then." To myself I added, "She'll see to that."

Those two weeks just slipped by. Mr. Allard was a whiz. He fixed my leaking hose and repaired my broken steps. He even replaced a bottom section of three logs in my sagging old house. That was a job and it took two. We used sturdy branches as levers, but it was sweat and strain more than anything else that got those logs in place. Mama was no help. In fact, she was a problem, determined to do her share.

"You stay back," I threatened her, "or so help me, I'll tie you to a tree."

I did let her help gather moss, which we used to chink in between the logs. There was much laughing and shouting and singing, not appreciated by certain of my friends. Minniebelle took off in disgust, hiding somewhere in the bush, pouting, I was sure. The mink no longer played on the beach and dragged their catch to my feet. The crows screeched their disapproval of the invasion, but I didn't care. In my affections Mama had replaced them all.

So far as Mr. Allard was concerned, Mama could do no wrong. Sometimes I suspected he even encouraged her in her mischief, though she didn't need it. They were in cahoots, those two, as I discovered one day when Mama took me aside.

"You could marry Mr. Allard, you know," she said.

I looked at her warily, wondering just how much scheming had actually gone on. She waited for me to speak, but I didn't. If she thought I was going to help her in this, she was mistaken. I looked as stern as I knew how, but it didn't dissuade her.

"You need a man around here," she reproached me. "Mr. Allard's a very nice man. I like him."

"I see that you do," I retorted, "but I'm the one that would have to live with him. If you don't mind, I'll just manage things my way."

For a while Mama was difficult, pursing her lips and shaking her head in disapproval every time she looked at me, but then Vera and Pat came in and everything was back on an even keel. They came, ostensibly, to bring me a salmon they just happened to catch, but in reality to hear more of Mama's jokes. She didn't disappoint them.

I was sorry that evening when Slim came to take Mama and Mr. Allard away. As I sat in my skiff, watching their boat disappear in the distance, I suddenly felt very lonely. All the laughter had gone from my cove. I turned to row back to the house, for no reason at all staring thoughtfully down into the water. Then I blinked in amazement, stopped my rowing, staring with mounting excitement into water that appeared to be black. Were my eyes deceiving me? No, it was true. I was floating in a swirling mass of millions of tiny black fish.

"Herring! They must be herring."

I let my boat drift. Not the slightest ripple betrayed my presence. The fish became playful, and I sat spellbound as they leaped all around me, the tinkle as their bodies struck the water like music in the night. I thrilled to the silver flashes of their bellies, like tiny lights in the dark. I was back in my own world, content.

Chapter 41

Mama must have taken the sunshine with her, I reflected one evening soon after she'd left, as I watched the fog creep in. It blanketed my world in a stillness so profound even the persistent ticking of the clock, when I retreated to the house, seemed muffled and indistinct. My world had closed in on me.

But in the night the stillness was broken, just a whisper at first, a gentle pattering of rain. Like music, its soft low undertones increased in a crescendo, the staccato tapping on my roof like the wild beat of native drums. Gradually the crescendo increased to a deafening roar. It was no longer possible to distinguish each separate beat. As I lay, wide-eyed and snug in my bed, I felt myself magically transported to a protected niche beneath some cascading waterfall. This noisy outpouring of nature, shattering the serenity of my tiny room, invaded my very being. As the roaring subsided, sleep came again.

The new day made a stealthy approach, for though the storm had abated, the clouds remained. The muted rumble of my waterfall so blended and harmonized that I was barely conscious of the sound. The gray waters of the sea, calm after the storm, now offered an irresistible invitation.

"Minniebelle!" I called, peeking into the bushes where she had taken refuge from the storm. "I'm going out in the boat."

A rustling in the bushes revealed her hiding place. She eyed me with what I took to be a look of disgust.

"I don't care," I defied her. "I *am* going."

It wasn't that easy. My boat, when I hauled it in, was half full of water. Anchored out in the cove, it had been a handy receptacle for the water that had been dumped from the skies onto my cove. It took a lot of bailing, but finally I was in my boat and headed for the waters beyond my islands, waters that, since Mama's coming, no longer intimidated me. I dipped my oars silently, reluctant to disturb the ethereal stillness of the day. Dark clouds heavy with the threat of more rain glowered over me, but for the moment there was a serenity, an empyreal hush that stirred the soul. My very aloneness was exciting, exhilarating.

As I sat quietly in my boat, I became aware of a presence. Mama had said it was not good that I should be alone in my wilderness home, but I knew that when I explained this moment to her, she would be satisfied. She would understand that I truly belonged here.

Slowly I turned and rowed back to my sheltered shores. The green of the forest, intensified by the drenching it had received, cast an eerie hue, deep, mysterious, almost somber, sustaining my solemn reflections. But the spell it cast was broken by the trilling song of a bird somewhere back in the bushes, and Minniebelle appeared, strutting saucily down the path ahead of me, looking back to make sure I was following.

"I'm coming, Minniebelle," I reassured her. "It will take more than a little rain to chase me away."

Will you try to live here?

The crackling fire in my old wood range was cheery and reassuring, overriding the persistent ping of stray raindrops in the pans I'd set out. That moment of doubt yielded to other concerns.

I had climbed up on the roof, shoving shingles into places where the leaks appeared to be, and they did stop some of the leaks, but in time the rain forced new passages through the old, eroded shingles that covered my kitchen roof.

Every day I faithfully bailed my skiff, more a matter of necessity than an act of love. The amount of rain that poured from the skies would most surely have sent one hapless boat to the bottom had I not persisted in my efforts. So I kept at it, wet as the day. I could as well be a duck, I thought, except a duck really was better endowed than I to keep dry. In spite of the rain, I went rowing out around my islands. I liked the feeling of the rain on my cheeks.

For nearly a week it rained steadily. My mail day arrived, but Slim failed to appear. I felt more concern over his failure to appear than over my need for food. Nevertheless, I started counting the days and counting my few remaining supplies.

There were still red berries on my bushes, and the goose-tongue on my beach was tender and green. On a low, low tide there would be clams for the taking, and the sea was full of fish if only I had the courage to go after them.

"Well, why not?" I demanded of myself. I'd fished plenty of times with Wally. I knew how. I knew the reefs where the snapper hung around. There was no reason I shouldn't get me a fish.

I hadn't forgotten the technique, but I sat for over an hour out there in the inlet while the rain trickled under the collar of my jacket and on down my neck.

I jigged with the persistence of a born fisherman, letting the line slip slowly through my fingers until it hit bottom, jerking it up quickly to give my lure the proper motion in the water, dropping it again . . . and again, patiently, tirelessly. Then at last, that jerk on the line, no mistake! Curbing my impatience, I reeled in slowly, just enough tension on the line. I could see him now, struggling to be free of the hook. I mustn't lose him. I wouldn't. I drew him up alongside the boat, reached for my gaff, and hit him over the head. Quickly I inserted the hook just below the head and lifted my fish into the boat. It was a beautiful red snapper .

I took my fish up with me even though I intended to fillet it on the beach. An overly curious mink or a greedy sea gull could steal my prize while my back was turned. Back on the beach, I selected a large flat rock and placed the snapper on it. From a short distance away a couple of sea gulls watched with covetous eyes.

I turned my attention back to my fish. Cleaning a salmon was easy, I reflected. You simply cut down the median line of the belly and stripped out the guts. But a snapper was different. It had a large bony cavern for its internal organs. Properly, the flesh must be cut from the bony structure without cutting into the bone. Tentatively, I stuck my knife in just below the head. Good! No bone. I slid my knife up, following the contour of the fleshy side, around, down toward the tail, and back up to my original cut. Now, if I could just slip my knife under and cut away from the bone. Ah, success!

One day I didn't row out, for the wind whipped through with relentless fury. Trees, swayed by the force of the wind, bent double, and an occasional crash in the forest told me some mighty giant had been toppled. The howl of the wind, the pounding of the sea, combined in a thunderous explosion. I'd stay inside if I had any sense, I told myself, but my nature rebelled. I stood on the beach, watching whitecapped waves march in as precisely as soldiers to battle. I thrilled at the resounding crash as they hit the shore and then, with a hissing and sucking, gave way to the next wave. I laughed at my gulls, huddled behind a log, seeking what little protection it afforded. No noisy interference this day!

The fury of the storm was matched by the swiftness of its passage, and I was left with the gentle rain. Almost two weeks since Slim had been in, two weeks without even a glimpse of a boat in the distance. I no longer listened for a friendly hum on the water. Then one day, as I stood at the sink, dodging stray raindrops while I washed my dishes, I heard the definite hum of an engine above the crackle of my fire. Hatless, coatless, I ran to the beach. It was Slim. I climbed in my boat and rowed out.

Slim laughed when he saw me. "You haven't improved, have you? No hat, no coat. I give up. You just don't listen."

"I was in a hurry."

"Aren't you always!" he chuckled. "Can't say as I blame you this time. Had a little trouble with my engine. Had to send out for a part. Hope you didn't run too short on supplies. Take my advice and order a little extra each time just in case something like this happens again."

Slim's visit made the day seem right. Though the rains continued, I really didn't mind. I had mail, letters from Mama and from Maureen and from my sister, Berne, in California. I also had food.

Chapter 42

One morning a peculiar brightness awakened me. I dressed hurriedly and ran out to see the mountains freed from their gray shackles. The sea glistened and shimmered as millions of dancing sunbeam sprites merrily stirred up the waters. Silver droplets of rain still clung to the maple leaves as though they had only been hung up to dry. A huge spiderweb, not yet dried by the sun, was a treasure chest of rainbow-hued jewels. Bees hummed as flowers lifted their heads to the sun. Minniebelle stomped purposefully down the path. The squirrels scampered through the filbert trees, and the mink claimed the beach. All around me in the bush were chirpings and twitterings. The birds were all singing, and there was an answering song in my heart.

I roamed the beaches looking for shells and drift. I wandered along my forest trails picking berries, and later in the day I made jelly from the berries I'd picked. The jelly would be good. I recalled a time Dr. and Mrs. McLean had stopped in for a quick cup of coffee with Wally and me. I'd served some of my jelly then.

"What kind of jelly is this?" Dr. McLean had asked.

"No special kind," I'd replied. "I just throw all kinds of berries in together. No recipe."

"Whatever," he said, "I've never tasted anything so good."

I'd given him a glass of jelly to take home. He was delighted.

And if he came again some time soon now I'd give him another glass, freshly made.

One beautiful day followed another. It was as if a repentant Mother Nature were trying to make amends for that long wet siege I'd had to endure. I cut wood sporadically, needing a hot fire only when I wanted to make more jelly. I took long walks and I picnicked on the beach and it didn't seem particularly wrong to just sit and do nothing, to idly watch a few stray clouds chasing each other across the limitless blue of the sky, to picture scenes in those clouds, a fluffy white lamb out to pasture, a puppy floating by on a downy bed, a rooster, head high as if crowing in triumph. What the eye can see!

And in the evenings, after I lit my lamp, I sat at the kitchen table making sea scenes from the shells and drift I'd collected. I fashioned seashell ladies and stood them on the top of my cupboards, and they kept me company.

Slim's next visit was a surprise. I'd lost track of the days. I'd forgotten to expect him. He grinned as I belatedly pulled up alongside the *Misty Lady*.

"You know," he said, "I had some reservations at first, about your staying way out here by yourself, but, by golly, I believe you're the happiest person I know."

"You'd better believe it," I retorted, grinning back at him.

The day after Slim's visit I was again running the beach, free as the wind, not a care, when of a sudden I felt a sharp pain in my foot. I sat down and removed my shoe, doubling myself into a knot as I examined every inch of my foot. There was no sign of a cut as from a broken clamshell, not even a prick, and no welt from a bite.

But when I came back in my foot was red and swollen. I tried to stand, but the pressure was intolerable. Hopping, hobbling, down on my knees on the steps, I made my way up to the house. Again I examined my foot. There was nothing to see, but my foot was throbbing now, radiating an intense heat. I could feel that heat on the palm of my hand without even touching my foot. Something must have poisoned me, but what? Could it have been one of those thousands of tiny transparent jellyfish that had floated in on the tide? Were they even poisonous? I wasn't sure, and I was too woozy to try to figure it out. The sensible thing would be to soak my foot in a solution of soda and go on up to bed. By morning it would surely be better.

I slept very little. The throbbing became a steady pound. Morning merely confirmed a suspicion that my condition had worsened. My ankle was now also red and swollen, and angry red streaks ran up my leg. Probably, I thought, I should go to the hospital at Esperanza. I realized that wasn't possible. Slim wouldn't be back for nearly a week. But there had to be something I could do. Maybe if I could get down to the beach I could signal a boat if one happened along.

Getting to the beach was more of a trial than I'd anticipated. I finally sat down on the steps and scooted from one to the other, but the jar as I landed on each step sent fresh stabs of pain coursing up my leg. I was glad to just sit on a rock on the beach, dabbling my feet in the water. Salt water was supposed to be healing. Maybe it would help me now. I sat for an interminable time, trying not to wonder what might become of me. I prayed for a boat, but no boat came. It was a lead-pipe cinch, Mama's expression, that if anything was to help me, it would still have to be something I could do for myself.

I made my way back to the house, where I elevated my leg and tried to think of every home remedy I'd ever known. Most of them I discarded as impractical, either because I didn't have the necessary ingredients or because they didn't pertain to my problem. The red streaks reached to my knee now. I made a soda paste and smeared it over my leg.

Morning came and I opened my eyes.

I did feel better. That queasy feeling in my stomach was gone. My foot was still swollen and feverish, but the red streaks had not advanced.

It was several days before I could bear weight on that foot, days in which I resented the confinement, but nonetheless I was buoyed by a sense of accomplishment. I was glad I hadn't gone to the hospital. Perversely, I forgot I had not had any choice.

Chapter 43

It had been so long since I'd had visitors. Except for those fifteen-minute intervals when Slim came in with mail and supplies, I'd been altogether alone ever since Mama left. The men were all fishing, and I watched their trollers go by, into Zeballos or Tahsis for supplies or repairs, back out to the open waters for another day's fishing. Life deals a strange hand, I thought. When my foot had threatened to put an end to my idyllic sojourn and I'd prayed for a boat, not one had appeared. Now there were many, any one of which, more than likely, I could signal, for all the good it would do. Too well I remembered that when Wally had died my signals went unnoticed.

I picked up a few stones and pegged them into the water, concentrating on the widening circles that marked their passage to the bottom of the cove, hoping thus to dispel thoughts that could only be distressful. If I was to stay on here, my thoughts must sustain, not shatter. The whine of a motor distracted me, and I looked to see where it was going.

"It seems to be coming here," I observed aloud.

Overcome by curiosity, I watched its approach. It was no troller. There were no lines, and it was too large. Then I recognized it—the Fisheries boat. But why was it coming to my cove? I waited for it to anchor off my islands, but it merely slowed down and kept moving in.

"You're crazy, whoever you are running that boat," I mumbled to myself. "You'll hang yourself up on my reefs."

Then I spotted a man kneeling on the prow, searching the water, signaling directions to the one who was steering. I held my breath as they zigzagged past my reefs until there they were . . . right in my harbor.

"You took an awful chance," I shouted. Then I blinked. "Dirk! Is that you?"

He grinned in reply. "Who else?"

Dirk belonged on the *Uchuck*. He was one of the crew. "What are you doing out here?" I demanded.

"Checking up on you! I have the day off and Jack has the afternoon free. What better way to spend the time? Are you going to ask us to come in?"

"Sure. I'll make you some coffee. Have you had lunch?"

"We have, but we'll take the coffee. By the way, this is Jack Fournier."

Jack had been setting the anchor, but now he bowed low. "About time you make the introductions, Mr. Kirkwood."

They were young, in their early twenties. There was a casual air about both that was engaging.

"Who helps you with your work?" Dirk asked some minutes later as we sat around the kitchen table drinking the coffee I'd brewed.

"I had a man in once to do the heavier work, but most things I do myself."

"Looks like maybe we'd better adopt you, eh, Mom?" A rakish grin accompanied Dirk's suggestion.

"So young," I thought, "so sure of himself." But with that curly black hair, the deep dimple in his chin, an Irish look, most surely he was the kind of boy Wally would have chosen as a son. We'd talked, sometimes, of adopting a boy, but it had gotten no further. Sad, I thought now, that when the boy we'd both wanted suddenly became reality, Wally wasn't here to share my delight.

"Suits me," I said. With the words came a sudden poignant realization that living here could be an even happier experience if someone really cared I was here.

"Come on, Mom, put us to work," Dirk said.

"Really! There's nothing to do." I answered.

"Sure there is. Where's your woodpile?"

I couldn't have stopped them had I wanted to. Never had I seen pieces of wood fly so fast. Best of all, they liked what they were doing.

"How about coming beachcombing with us?" Jack asked when they were finished. "We'll head out to Catala Island. Should be a lot of loot on the outer beaches."

"I'd love it. You know, I've been here nearly four months now and the only time I've been off this place was when I went on the *Uchuck* to Ferrier, and there I never set foot on land. It'll be fun tramping along some beach other than my own."

Catala fronted on an unlimited expanse of ocean. Anchoring on the leeward side, we rowed to shore, stashing our skiff well above the high-tide line. Then, each with a gunny sack slung over our shoulders, we worked our way over the rocky ledges to the outside beach. We raced along the beach, climbed over logs, calling out over each new find. The sacks became heavy with their burden of glass balls, pieces of driftwood, shells of all description, loot so precious we disregarded the stench of decaying bodies in some of the shells and the salty smell of drift washed again and again by the waters that surged in from the sea.

Dirk laughed as he spoke to me: "By the time you get home you're going to smell like some old dead fish."

"So!" I shrugged the words away. No concern about a dead-fish smell was going to spoil my day.

We should have been satisfied with what we had gathered so far, but, contemplating treasures that might be found beyond a cliff, we decided to scale it. It was steep, jagged. The boys started their climb, and I followed, not far behind. Digging my toes into a crevice, I reached for a handhold and then another. I even dared an occasional glance at the sea thundering below me. It hurled itself against the rocky barricade, threatening to hurdle it. Spray filled the air, droplets falling over my shoulders. Fascinated, I continued to climb. The boys stopped and looked back, and they grinned.

"Come on, Mom. Don't hold up the parade."

I liked that. They gave me credit for being able to make my own way. It was not like being a woman and two boys. We were just three people having fun.

Another sandy beach stretched out on the far side of the cliff. Jack pointed excitedly to a tiny peninsula where three deer—a buck, a doe, and a fawn—were grazing. He ran to flush them while Dirk and I concealed ourselves at the foot of a ledge where they were almost certain to pass. We were not disappointed. The buck leaped over the ledge, dropping almost at my feet. I quivered with delight, hardly daring to breathe. He stood poised for a moment, head held high, nostrils quivering, then bounded into the brush, the doe and the fawn close at his heels.

"Gosh, Dirk," I whispered, still under the spell. "I've never been so close to a buck. I could have reached out and touched him."

We selected a log and sat watching the sun beat a blazing retreat into the sea. Then, nursing our sacks of loot, we made our way back to our skiff. It was dark before we reached it, and out over the black waters our ship was barely discernible.

It was good to be back on board. I offered to help prepare supper but was relieved when my offer was rejected.

"No room for three to work in this galley, Mom. You take it easy. Climb up on that bunk there and relax. You'll see. We're passable cooks."

They were. The meal was excellent, ham and potatoes, string beans, even a salad, and what a treat to be served.

Time then to haul anchor. As we ventured out, the reflections of millions of stars winked up at us. Our ship parted the waters, leaving in our wake a fantail of silvery spray. In the distance my islands assumed a ghostlike appearance. We cut our speed, cautious on approach. In the dark those reefs were more formidable.

"Don't try to go in," I said.

So they lowered the skiff. Dirk jumped down into it, and I followed. A few deft strokes and I was back on my own shores. I stood there a moment watching the boat steal away in the darkness. Then I turned and looked up at my house, dark and quiet and empty.

Chapter 44

The shortening August days were lazy and relaxing. During the morning hours the sun picked up moisture from the sea, returning it in the afternoon in the form of fog. It crept in silently, following the contour of the land, a low fog that clung to the sea, enhancing the sharpness of mountain peaks outlined against the sky. The fog clung mainly to the north shore. While looking out on a spectacular sight, that billowing mass of white against a background of forest green, I still basked in the sun.

There was life all about . . . the wind whispering through the trees, the brush of a wing as a bird darted by, the skittering in the bushes of some friendly creature, and, as I lay there on the beach, my ear pressed close to the ground, the fascinating sounds of the sea, tiny crabs and snails moving and stirring.

It seemed people were determined to come. I wasn't too surprised that Dirk and Jack came back. They brought me a salmon. No time this day for beachcombing, but they insisted they had time to chop wood.

"Someone's got to look after you, Mom," Dirk declared. "Who better than us?"

Who better indeed! Not that I felt I needed looking after, but they were so gloriously young. When they came the cove seemed to take on new dimensions.

With Joan and Bill it was different. I had wished all sum-

mer I could see them, but I hadn't expected them. I knew Bill
fished long, hard hours, hours that didn't leave time for much
else. But I couldn't forget that when Wally and I came to the
cove Bill had been our first client. We hadn't planned on
practicing veterinary medicine here on the island, but a visit
from Bill with four Airedale pups to be spayed had changed
that.

So the day I saw *Maggie* heading for the cove I was really
excited. *Maggie* was still painted the leaded orange color I had
found so pleasing. I couldn't mistake her, set apart by her
color from the traditionally white trollers that passed by the
cove.

Bill hadn't changed, either. He was as lean as ever. His
Adam's apple still ran up and down his throat when he laughed
the easy, comfortable laughter that accompanied almost every
statement he made. While Joan selected flat rocks and spread
out the contents of the picnic basket she'd brought, Bill
lounged on the beach, arranging his long body on the rocks in
such a way that the rocks seemed more to be props than
obstacles.

"We didn't mean to neglect you," Joan said, "but with Bill
away fishing all summer . . . I never see him. I could as well
be a wid—" She stopped and bit her lip.

"It's okay, Joan," I replied quickly. "I've had a beautiful
summer, truly I have."

Joan shook her head, half doubting my words. "Well,
maybe," she conceded, "but surely the summer must have
shown you that you can't stay on here."

"Wrong, Joan. Oh, I can't stay this winter. I know that.
Slim said there might be weeks at a time when he wouldn't
be able to get out. But come spring, I'll be back."

Joan opened her mouth to speak, but Bill got his words in
first. "Come off it, Joaney. She knows what she can do." His
good-natured laugh broke the tension, leading us into more
casual talk as we gathered around Joan's improvised picnic
table.

When Frank and Eva came out from Zeballos, my suspicion
that local people felt I wouldn't be returning was confirmed.

Wally and I had removed a tumor from the leg of Hank's old springer on one of our trips into Zeballos. Hank and Eva had thought a lot of Doc, as they called him, but never once, while Wally was alive, had they been out to the cove. They'd been meaning to come all summer, they told me, wanting to see me before I left. They planned now to stay but a couple of hours—they shouldn't be away from their hardware store in Zeballos too long, they insisted at first—but somehow their stay lengthened to two days.

"Do you mind?" they asked. "It's so wonderfully peaceful here. Let them bang on our door in Zeballos. They can wait."

Dr. and Mrs. McLean came from their mission hospital at Esperanza, "just for a cup of coffee and some of your good jelly." They stayed the night.

"I'm sure there's nothing right now the nurses can't handle. Here, there's such a feeling of serenity. No room for tensions." Dr. McLean leaned back in Wally's rocker, a smile easing the tired lines of his face. No suggestion from them that I wouldn't be back, and I realized then how much Dr. McLean must have loved the cottage across the cove, what it must have cost him to give it up, to sell it to us, though recognizing his place was in Esperanza.

My cove, I could see, had become a place of refuge for others as well as for me. I liked having company, yet, coming so late in the summer, it disturbed me. I rejected any reminder that the time was approaching when I must leave. And as for not coming back! Well, they would see.

The fog that had plagued the far shore in the late afternoon had slipped on across the inlet, blanketing the sea one night. Under this blanket sounds were held down, magnified, and then I heard voices. Had someone, in the dark, confused by the fog, wandered onto my reefs? My flashlight beam barely pierced the mists as I felt my way over the boulders to the outside beach. All I could see of the boat was the blur of its lights. The engine was silent. Then I heard a splash as the anchor was dropped, and as I strained to see, a small skiff took shape, indistinct, ghostlike in the wavering mists.

"Mrs. Flynn! Are you all right?" It was Rose's voice, and

as they approached I could see Alban was with her, also five of their children, all crowded into that one small boat.

I laughed with relief. "I'm fine. I heard voices and thought someone had stumbled on my reefs."

Alban shook his head. "No. We know your reefs."

"Thank heaven!" I replied. "Since you're all here, why don't you come up to the house? I could fix us a snack. Seems so long since I've seen you."

"We'll come," Rose decided. "We want to see you, but Alban's been fishing. All our men fish except Pat. Now Pat, he's working at a logging camp, so we have no boat at our village. Today Alban say, 'We will go to Zeballos. Is time to buy clothes for the kids.' They will go back to school soon," Rose explained.

"Whatever brought you this way, I'm happy," I said as I led the way up the steps.

I was happy also that my Indian neighbors were never in a hurry. They stayed several hours. When we ventured back into the night, the fog had slipped on up the inlet toward Zeballos, leaving our area in the clear. With an untroubled mind I watched as their boat glided away on a moonlight trail.

One day, again, I had a visitor. This man confessed, quite bluntly, that he had come because he was curious.

"I just don't believe any woman would really want to live alone way out here. How old are you anyway?"

Amused, I tried to recall the five ages Wally had claimed were peculiar to each individual. I wasn't sure I had them right, but I gave them to him the way I remembered them.

"Well, let's see. There's a hereditary age, a biological age, a psychological age, a physiological age, and, less important, but the one everyone seems most concerned about, the chronological age. Go ahead. Take your pick."

To these five ages I could have added a sixth, an environmental age, for here in the bush, exposed to clean air, with exercise a part of living, the body loses excess pounds, muscles firm, the skin glows, and one's step is light and firm. I saw that my guest studied me speculatively. A twinkle in his eyes suggested he had picked an age.

We chatted for a while. Rather, he asked questions, and I answered them as I saw fit.

Then, quite abruptly, he stated, "I'm disappointed."

Such an outright declaration was startling. "In what way?" I demanded.

"You're normal!" was the unexpected rejoinder. "You aren't eccentric." And with a sort of begrudging admiration, he added, "You're even intelligent."

I was convulsed with laughter. After a moment's hesitation, he joined in. "I'll give you three years here," he said. "By then you'll have your bellyful of it."

Chapter 45

Yellow leaves on my maple, like pieces of gold, announced the arrival of September. Mountain ash was a startling combination of red and black. The brightness of the berries was offset by the somber black dress of the crows who had deserted my clam beds for easier picking in the ash.

"You're drunk," I challenged them, watching their skitterish maneuverings. "Don't you know those overripe berries are like aged wine?"

If they knew, they didn't care, too content or too surfeited to emit even the familiar caw. My blue jays, however, made up for the lessened belligerence of my crows. Their strident voices mingled with the chattering of the squirrels as they quarreled over my ripening nuts. Occasionally a jay would jab his beak too far into a nut.

"That should silence you for a while." And I watched in amusement as the disgruntled jay pounded the nut against the trunk of a tree or on the roof of the house until the nut split, freeing his beak.

Minniebelle held herself aloof from all of this, quarreling with no one, satisfied to nibble at the greengage plums that festooned the side of the house.

It was a happy scene, all of it, yet I couldn't escape a feeling of sadness. Could it be because I planned to leave at the end of September? The number of my visitors, the unmistakable signs of fall, had made me cognizant of the passage of time. During the past months a week between Slim's visits had often seemed long. Now a month, as I contemplated leaving, seemed no time at all. Maybe I could shake the feeling by clearing a trail to my blackberry patch. I hacked for hours at the tangled growth, too tired at the end to be sad.

The berries were plump and juicy, but I paused before plunging into the patch. Bears liked berries, too. None seemed to be present at the moment, but I had no doubts I'd be sharing that patch.

One day I danced with excitement. I'd heard the familiar drone of the plane before I saw it. I couldn't be mistaken. The drone of that engine, those years Wally and I flew the coast, had become a part of me, my ears attuned to its monotony, alert to any change that could indicate trouble. That was our plane, I decided now, and it was coming my way.

Last fall, after Wally's death, I'd offered the plane to Father Lobsinger. He deserved it, I felt, for it was he who had sent us to this cove. I knew, also, the priests' need of a plane. Visting all the Indian villages along the hundred-mile stretch of coast that extended from Christie, their mission boarding school on Meares Island, north to the village of Kyuquot was a long and hazardous journey by boat. A plane, taking advantage of favorable weather, could transport them speedily from one village to another.

My decision to give the plane to the priests hadn't been altogether altruistic, however. I wanted that plane up there in the skies, flying the route Wally and I knew so well. How better than in the hands of the priests? Our pigeon had not been a pleasure craft, but had taken us safely to all those places where we carried on our practice of veterinary medicine. With the priests she would be working still.

"A plane would be an answer to prayer," Father Lobsinger had assured me. "But are you sure that's what you want to do with it?"

I was sure, but giving a plane away wasn't all that easy, I discovered. The plane wasn't legally mine to do anything with until the terms of Wally's will had been satisfied. Transferring ownership from one country to another presented more legal problems. Canadian standards required certain changes on the plane itself, work which must be done before it could pass Canadian inspection. In the meantime, three of the priests had learned to fly. And now, at last, the yellow pigeon was back in the skies where she belonged.

And then I saw the yellow-and-maroon of our pigeon outlined against the blue of the skies, and the surge of joy that trembled my body was indescribable. No matter who held the title, in my heart that yellow pigeon would always be ours . . . Wally's and mine. As I waited in almost intolerable anticipation, the plane landed, taxied cautiously past our reefs and up onto the floating ramp Wally and I had worked so hard to build. The engine was silenced. The propeller made one final feeble flip. Then the doors were flung open and two men stepped down onto the pontoons.

"By heaven! It's good to see you!" Father Lobsinger did the speaking. "How are you?" Father Larkin waved his hand in greeting.

"I'm fine," I assured them, then added, "You landed and taxied in here like a veteran."

"I did all right then?" Father Lobsinger valued my praise, but he valued the plane more. "It's a great plane," he said.

Both men were in the process of pulling on hip boots. They waded to shore, then followed me up to the house, where I made coffee and sandwiches.

"Don't go to a lot of bother," Father Lobsinger insisted. "We're heading up to Kyuquot so can't stay long. We stopped in, really, to see how you've been making out, of course, but also to ask for your help."

I was puzzled, but made no comment, waiting for Father Lobsinger to continue.

"How would you like to come down to Christie School for a while?"

The question took me by surprise. I hesitated, pondering my answer. "I don't know," I said finally. "I fail to see what I could contribute. Are you sure you aren't asking me out of charity, thinking I'm lonely, or despondent? I'm not, you know."

There was a chuckle of appreciation from Father Lobsinger. Father Larkin laughed outright.

"Just like a woman," he said, "always suspecting an angle. But you're right. There is an angle, only to our benefit. You know, of course, that our staff is Indian. It's worked out fine in every department except the kitchen. They're good workers and excellent cooks, but they all want to be in charge, refuse to take orders from each other. It's chaos. We talked it over with them and they all agreed if you came down and supervised there'd be no more fighting."

"But I don't know a thing about running a kitchen," I protested, "and I'm no great shakes at keeping order, either. I'm not qualified."

"Sure you are," Father Lobsinger reiterated. "You already know several of the women, and even those you don't know hold you in pretty high regard. The Indian people feel that yellow plane sitting out there belongs to all of them, not just to the priests."

"Well, in a way I guess it does." I thought for a moment, considering the implications. "I guess I could try," I volunteered at last, "but I'm not guaranteeing the results."

"That's all we ask," Father Larkin contended. "How about today? We could pick you up on our way back from Kyuquot."

"Today?" It was a cry of dismay. What of my plans to stay here at the cove through September? "Oh, I couldn't," I protested. "The house has to be cleaned and in order before I leave for the winter. Besides, Slim will be in tomorrow. If I'm not here he'll imagine all kinds of things."

"Okay. We'll pick you up in four days then. How's that?"

Four days was nothing, but what could I say? "I'll be ready," I promised.

Chapter 46

"Well, that's a sorry state of affairs," Slim declared when I broke the news about going to Christie. "Making this run out here has gotten to be a habit. I'll miss it."

"Oh, I'll be back in the spring, Slim. You watch for me. By the way, do you think the store will take back the groceries I ordered for today? Seems I won't be needing them."

"I'll take them if they won't," Slim reassured me. "There's nothing in your order I can't use."

"Thanks, Slim. I've a big packet of letters for you to mail, too. I wrote everyone I know last night, telling them I was leaving here and going down to Christie."

There was an ache in my heart telling Slim good-bye. It was much more than saying good-bye to a friend. Without his help my summer would have fizzled. I stood on the beach, staring up the inlet long after his boat had disappeared from view.

I felt sad all that day and the next morning, too, as I went about my task of closing the house up for the winter. I wasn't ready to leave. This summer I hadn't just tried to live here. I'd wanted to live here. This was home. I was folding clothes in the afternoon and putting them away when I heard a shout from the beach.

"Mrs. Flynn! Mrs. Flynn!" The voice was clearly Indian, the *nn* in Flynn cut short, as if there were only one.

"Good!" I thought as I ran to the beach. "I'll be able to let them know at Nuchatlitz now that I'm leaving."

Frank and Sophie Savey were waiting patiently in their old dugout canoe.

"You sure sneak up on a person in that canoe," I greeted them, laughing.

"Ah, but it's good, this canoe. Outboards . . . they are for the young," Frank observed. "Paddles, they are more sure."

"And your canoe is more beautiful," I assured him.

"It is very old, old like us, but in this canoe, my wife and I, we feel safe. We would have come sooner to see you, but my heart . . . it is not good."

"But you're here now, and I'm glad. Won't you come up and have dinner with me?" It wasn't dinnertime, I reflected, but with the Indian people dinner could be served at any time of the day.

After dinner I suggested we pick blackberries. "I have a lovely patch. Now that I'm leaving I'll never be able to use all those berries."

"I'll wait in the canoe," Frank said. "My heart!"

So Sophie and I picked berries. She spoke no English, I spoke no Indian, but the words flowed between us. "Here's a good spot. Lots of berries here." There was an empathy that overcame the confusion of words. It gave me a warm happy feeling, and Frank's parting comment added to that feeling.

"Is good that you go to Christie, but you come back. Dr. Flynn, your husband, good to Nuchatlitz. Nuchatlitz take care of his wife."

The fourth day arrived and I was ready, though still unwilling. The day before, I'd taken my boat out of the water on the very highest tide. The priests could help me drag it into the bush. This morning I folded my bedding and put it in my storage chest. I turned off the outside water faucet so if the hose sprang a leak the whole creek wouldn't flow through my house. I took my leftover lettuce and cabbage down to the beach and tossed it to the gulls.

I laughed at their greedy endeavors to snatch bits from each other even while greens dangled from their own beaks.

I sat on the beach and watched, waiting until the sun sank over Mount Eliza, and yet no yellow pigeon appeared in the sky. I accepted it philosophically. I almost gloated—another day at the cove!

I went up to the house and turned on the water faucet. I built a fire in my stove and went upstairs and rolled out my sleeping bag. Then I looked in the pantry, debating what I should eat. The shelves looked rather bare, but there were still a few tins. I selected a couple and prepared a leisurely supper.

The next morning I repeated the procedure of the previous day, rolled up my sleeping bag, turned off the faucet, and went down to the beach to wait. It was a procedure I repeated for the next three days. I felt rather like a kid playing truant from school. It was a nice feeling.

Two more days passed. My supply of canned goods had all but disappeared, and Slim wouldn't be back to replenish it. I'd picked blackberries, but with the help of the birds and the bears, they were fast disappearing. I'd gathered clams on a low tide, but there wouldn't be another tide sufficiently low for maybe two weeks. If only I hadn't beached my boat on that highest tide, I could have gone fishing. I'd checked my tide book. There'd not be another tide all month high enough to float it.

Even disregarding my lack of food, I just plain missed the rowing. For the first time vague misgivings pricked at my placidity. How many days had I been waiting anyway? I tried to figure back. Must be close to a week, I decided. The priests had been delayed, perhaps by an emergency at school, or possibly there was a problem with the pigeon. The weather was perfect.

I sat down at the beach. A sea gull lit near me, snatched a fish from the water, and took off, several other gulls screaming in pursuit. I wished he'd drop that fish near me. I'd grab it. It began to rain, straight down, as if the sky had been rent with a giant knife, letting it all spill out. For sure the plane wouldn't come now. I was wet to the skin. I went back to the house.

It continued to rain, and I lost track of the days, but every day I bailed out my boat. Minniebelle had sought the cover of the brush, but she ventured out when I did, ruffling her feathers in greeting. I didn't linger long for a visit. This was a cold rain. I craved the warmth of my fire, and as I snuggled close I wished I hadn't been so thorough in cutting myself off . . . telling Slim and the Indians I was leaving . . . and all those letters I'd written. No one would feel any concern, taking it for granted I was busy at school, too busy to write more letters. It wasn't staying on that bothered me, even in the rain. What bothered me was that no one, except the priests, thought I was here, and maybe, in all this long time, even they had forgotten me. Or maybe they had simply decided they didn't want me.

Now, with more time on my hands, my active imagination took over. It *could* be possible they didn't want me at Christie. After a time I realized I was being ridiculous. The priests here on the coast had accepted us, had treated us like any other parishioners. How could I think they would reject me now? Then maybe they'd had an accident with the pigeon.

As I bailed my boat one day, a motion in the water caught my eye. I watched the widening circles, wondering.

"Oscar!" I cried, as a seal's head poked up out of the water. "Oh, am I glad to see you."

Oscar had come in often that last year Wally and I spent here together. His appearance now made me feel not so alone and forgotten. He swam all around, he dived and I tried to speculate where his head would reappear next. And then he came in close. I could swear he was grinning.

"You silly creature!" And I laughed. My depressed mood had vanished.

Oscar kept me company in the days that followed. I never knew just when to expect him, and as I didn't want to miss him, it entailed countless trips to the beach. His visits kept me occupied as nothing else could have. Chopping wood and bailing the boat were necessary chores, but they did nothing to halt the distressing thoughts that would creep in. With Oscar around I could think of nothing but Oscar. His antics were a delight to watch, his companionship a joy.

One day brought sunshine again. Its dazzling rays streaking through my rain-drenched evergreens sparked a new hope. Surely Father Lobsinger would come now. And after a while I did hear a hum, but it wasn't a plane. It was a boat. I turned away, kicking absentmindedly at some pebbles on the beach. I had heard boats before, had seen them, but they'd stayed close to Center Island, too far away to notice a signal even if I'd tried to send one, and anyway, from my experience when Wally had died, I knew they would be unlikely to look my way. Really, there was no reason to glance my way. No one was home, or so they thought. However, the hum increased in intensity. This boat surely wasn't hugging Center Island. Curious, I turned to look out over the inlet. I saw the boat then, close to my shores. It was coming in. I hardly dared let myself believe, but yes, it was coming in.

"Pat's boat! That's Pat's boat." I was laughing and crying at the same time, choking over the lump that filled my throat.

"Pat!"

"Mrs. Flynn!" We spoke in unison.

"Mrs. Flynn," Pat repeated, "I thought you were at Christie."

"They didn't come," I told him, and I was laughing, for how could I be downcast with Pat standing there in his boat grinning down at me? "How did you happen to come?" I demanded.

"I come to saw a log for you so you have plenty of wood when you come back. Many logs floating. I figure the storm would drive some in here. It did, too. That's a fir over there."

When you come back. Those words struck home. My Indian neighbors believed I would come back.

"Pat," I said at last, remembering I was not being a proper hostess. "I can't invite you to dinner. I have only crackers and peanut butter, and not much of that anymore."

"Today I can't stay." He answered as if my lack of food were not the reason at all. "I'll go now to Esperanza. I'll tell them to come."

The rest of the day passed as in a dream. I emptied my buckets and set them back in place for more rain that would surely come. I cleaned up the mess I'd made of my house, all the wet leaves and evergreen needles I'd tracked in. I let the fire die in the stove, scraped the ashes into the ash box and carried it out to the ash heap. And I sang as I worked. Tomorrow I would be leaving; Pat would see to it.

I was up early the next morning, watching. Pat hadn't come back. I hadn't expected him. He'd told me his mission. I should need no further assurance. I waited now for someone, anyone, from Esperanza. My ears were primed for the familiar hum, and when I heard it I raced to the farthest point of the beach so I could watch the boat as it approached. So great was my excitement that I could hardly maintain my balance on the rocky shore as I ran with the boat back into the cove.

"Mrs. Flynn!" That was Mrs. McLean's voice. "Oh, we're so sorry. We had no idea you were here all this time. The doctor and I will take you right to Esperanza. You can stay with us until the *Uchuck* goes out."

Dr. McLean tossed me his tie-down rope, and I looped it around a boulder. "Don't try to come ashore," I said. "I'll just grab my bags and wade out . . ."

The last words trailed off as I cocked my head, listening. "That's the plane," I shouted. "They're coming, too."

"What do you want to do?" Mrs. McLean asked.

"I don't know. I guess all I can do is wait and see if they still want me at Christie."

"We'll wait, too," Mrs. McLean said firmly. "I'm not leaving until you're either on that plane or here in the boat with us."

It was taking so long, I thought. Why didn't they hurry? And all the time I knew they couldn't, for my reefs could not be circled in a hurry. At last the pigeon was in the cove and up on the float. Father Lobsinger stepped down onto the pontoon.

"Well! A welcoming committee, or is it? I almost wondered if I dared come in." His usual self-assurance was missing.

"Oh, you're most welcome," I assured him, "though you just caught me. I was about to leave with the McLeans. Perhaps I still should, if you don't need me at Christie. Things have probably straightened themselves out by now."

"Afraid not. We still want you. I'm sorry about the delay. Had a little problem with the plane here. Couldn't get the part we needed in Vancouver. Had to send back east. Every day we thought for sure it would come. The days kept piling up. Twenty-two days since we promised to pick you up. By heaven, that's a long time."

To me it had seemed twice as long! I thanked the McLeans for coming, assured them I'd see them in the spring, then waded out to the pigeon, a bag in each hand.

"Tell me," Father Lobsinger said as he reached for a bag, "what did you really think of us all this long time you were alone?"

"Well, Father," and I grinned up at him as he held out a hand to pull me up onto the pontoon, "every day I said to myself, 'I'll give them just one more day!'"

Chapter 47

Sitting on the damp steps of my kitchen porch after a night of heavy rain, I thought back on the months I'd been away. I had wanted to get back to reassure myself I could still chop wood and cut brush, that life in the wilds still held its appeal. I looked up at Minniebelle, regarding me placidly from her perch in the plum tree. Playfully I bent to pick up a twig, tossing it in her direction. She chose to ignore it, too accustomed to me to be startled at whatever I might do. I laughed my delight, exulting in the closeness between us. I sniffed the air. Definitely, life in the wilds still held its appeal.

"Minniebelle," I said, "don't you ever desert me, not ever, as long as I come here, and I hope," I added, more to myself than to her, "that will be for many, many years."

Minniebelle nodded, and my mind wandered back to those days at Christie School after Father Lobsinger had finally picked me up from the cove here. It had been a drastic change from the cove . . . so much activity, with one hundred and fifty Indian children running up and down the halls of that rambling three-story building. The children, with their short-cropped black hair and their smiling dark brown eyes, were lovable and eager to know me. Father Noonan, the school principal, and the six Sister teachers all made me feel welcome. The Indian staff workers accepted me; they liked me. I'd decided I couldn't have found a happier place to spend the winter months.

Over and over I said to myself, "I love these people."

Actually, it was the children who nudged me into becoming a Catholic. I went with them to Mass, but I couldn't receive the sacraments, as they did. They didn't question me aloud, but their eyes said, "Why aren't you like us?"

I paused in my reflections and giggled, glancing up to see if Minniebelle was still with me, glad to see that she was.

"Minniebelle, you wouldn't believe the situations I can get into. I was so proud that first Sunday I attended Mass. I had a dress to wear. You've seen me wear it once or twice when I wanted to remind myself I was a lady. You know the one, that pretty yellow one with the full pleated skirt."

She ruffled her feathers and lifted her wings, evidently tired of sitting looking at me.

"No fair, Minniebelle," I cried. "I'm not through talking to you.

"Okay, stay put awhile. Well, I was confident I looked really great in that yellow dress, even though there was no mirror in my room to confirm it. They're funny about mirrors. Something about resisting vanity. I still don't understand. Anyway, I followed the children into the chapel. It's a lovely chapel, Minniebelle. Father Noonan told me later the altar and all the statues came by boat from Victoria. It can seat two hundred comfortably, and on this Sunday every seat was taken. The children and the Sisters sit in the front section. I sat with the staff, behind them, and behind us were the priests and several Brothers who work around the school. There were also some visiting priests."

I'd enjoyed Mass, kneeling and standing, taking my cue from the others. Sometimes it had seemed to me, when Wally and I had attended Mass together in times past, that Catholics were always bobbing up and down. I had never understood why, at a certain time, one must kneel or stand, but I'd conformed, as I did this day. One thing puzzled me greatly, however. As the Mass progressed, the priests and the Brothers, one by one, got up and left the chapel. I wondered what could be so urgent that it would take them all away from Mass. But after Mass I forgot all about it as I rushed down to the kitchen to see about preparations for the noon meal. I was swishing around, feeling important, when a sixth-grade Indian girl came up to me.

"Mrs. Flynn!" she exclaimed. "Did you go to Mass like that?"

I stared at her, bewildered. Didn't I look beautiful? Then Sister Amelia came up and started to laugh. The entire back of my dress was caught up in my belt. Every time I'd bobbed at Mass I'd presented the priests and the Brothers with a full view of my undergarments. No wonder they had all left the chapel.

"They shouldn't have looked," Sister Amelia declared, still laughing. "They're always telling women they shouldn't be looking around noticing what others are wearing. Serves them right."

It wasn't funny. I retreated to a table in the farthest corner of the kitchen, hoping no one would notice me, but Father Noonan did. My skirt was now where it belonged, but his blue eyes had a mischievous glint. There was an unnatural flush on his cheeks, and as he rocked back and forth, heel to toe, there was a suspicious quirk at the corners of his mouth. I knew he wanted to laugh, but he merely nodded and went on.

"Stop hiding," Sister Amelia urged me a few minutes later. "No one thinks anything about it."

"I'm sure!" I retorted. "Why did they all leave then?" And I groaned. "Poor Brother Ed! He was right behind me. It must have been awful for him."

"He probably couldn't care less."

"Just the same, I'm not going to Mass next Sunday."

Sister Amelia scolded me after that Mass. "You could just as well have come. Brother Ed wasn't there either."

I laughed, thinking about it now, then got up and ran down to the beach, where I could bask in the sun. It was chilly sitting on that damp step, and so long as Minniebelle wasn't going to hang around, there was no sensible reason to sit there

soaking up dampness. It was pleasant on the beach. I wandered
around a bit looking to see if the night tide had brought in
anything interesting. It hadn't, so I settled myself on a large
flat boulder, my thoughts still on Christie.

Brother Ed and I had both soon recovered from our em-
barrassment. If the incident wasn't forgotten, it was shelved.
I was more concerned about that question in the children's
eyes. "Why aren't you like us?" I went to Father Noonan and
told him I'd like to become a Catholic. Instruction was
started immediately.

One evening, when I'd been at Christie a little over a
month, I was sitting on the counter in the kitchen watching
some of the older girls scrub the floor. Father Noonan was
standing beside me. We had been laughing and joking, but of
a sudden I felt a prickling sensation at the base of my skull.
I frowned, turning my head slightly from side to side.

"Something wrong?" Father Noonan asked.

"I don't know." I paused, turned my head to the side again.
"My neck seems to be stiff, and I have a tingling feeling all
down my spine. Oh, I'll be all right. I'll just go on up to bed."
I slid off the counter and, disregarding his puzzled frown,
climbed the stairs to my room.

Morning came and I didn't get up. What was the matter
with me? Sister Amelia came in to see why I hadn't come
down to the kitchen.

"I can't move," I told her. My eyes must surely have reflected my fright, my feeling of utter helplessness. "I can't
turn over. I can't even feel my arms or my legs."

"Lie still," she said. As if I could do anything else! "I'll go
get Father Noonan."

Father Noonan sent for the doctor at Tofino. He was young
and he wanted to help. He took my legs, bending them at the
knee, back and forth, and did the same with my arms. He took
my hands, manipulating each finger, but no feeling came.

"It's hard to say what it is," he said. "It acts somewhat
like acute arthritis, but I'm not sure. It could be psycho-
somatic. Sometimes shock will trigger something like this,

even delayed shock. It's only been a little over a year since you lost your husband. You've had to make a lot of radical adjustments. I don't want to frighten you now, but I must be honest. Sometimes a condition like this gets progressively worse."

I cried after he left. A cripple for the rest of my life! Unable to go back to the cove! I'd rather be dead.

I could hear the footsteps of the children as they ran up and down the long hall. I could hear a thud in the playroom above me when some heavy object was dropped on the floor. I could hear the scraping of chairs and the happy sound of laughter.

Daily I grew more depressed, more frightened. I hated my room and I hated the school. Most of all, I hated myself. I had come here to help these people. Now they had to help me. It was humiliating. I turned in upon myself, trying to shut out those who would help me, wallowing in a plethora of self-pity and sheer terror.

"It's no use, Father," I said to Father Noonan. "The doctor's been here almost every day for over a week now. He says I may never walk again. I can't take instruction. I can't read. I can't even think."

"You can think," he said sternly. "You're just thinking the wrong thoughts. When you're over this we'll continue your instruction."

His attitude shocked me, then started me thinking. I'd been miserable, totally, thoroughly miserable, to everyone who'd tried to help me. I hadn't cooperated, not with them, not with the doctor. I'd let him manipulate my arms and legs, but had made no effort to try for myself. I'd been content to just lie back and suffer. What an absolutely disgusting creature I'd become. Tears filled my eyes, but I willed them away. Enough of self-pity!

Later that day those feet pounding down the long hall stopped at my door. The door swung open, revealing the eager faces of some of my little Indian friends. Their round, velvety brown eyes regarded me solemnly.

"Can you walk yet, Mrs. Flynn? We prayed for you."

That was more than I'd done for myself, and I was ashamed. They came often after that, bringing pictures they'd drawn, colorful sketches of life as they saw it.

"We'll put them on the wall for you, Mrs. Flynn. Then you can see them."

Soon my walls were covered with pictures. It was impossible to be glum with so much love and happiness surrounding me. My resentment vanished without my even realizing it. Somehow it just wasn't there anymore. And then Sister Ruth Ann came with a suggestion.

"The third- and fourth-graders would like to teach you your catechism, if you wouldn't mind."

Mind? It was like throwing a life preserver to a drowning person. It could keep my mind occupied, keep it off myself. And so they came, after their classes were over for the day, reading to me from the instruction book, slow, halting words, asking the questions, bright eyes anticipating my answers. Then a giggle.

"No, Mrs. Flynn. Guess again."

"I'll help you, Mrs. Flynn. It says . . . Now can you say the rest?"

I looked forward to those after-school sessions when my happy young instructors piled into my room. With so many, there was bound to be confusion. Often there was more giggling than teaching, but I concentrated between the giggles, determined my young teachers should be proud of me. Father Noonan grinned his approval when he came in one day.

"We'll make you a Catholic yet," he said.

My spirits were good. I could even wiggle around a bit, though my arms and legs refused to function. My doctor voiced his concern.

"We're not getting you on your feet. I think maybe we should send you to a specialist in Vancouver."

"Oh, please, no!" I begged. "Give me another week here anyway. Maybe something will happen."

He shook his head, but agreed to the week. After he left I thought for a long time. I remembered myself running down the stairs with a number of the children.

"Are you young or old?" one of them had demanded.

I had paused, considering. "That's a hard question to answer," I said finally. "It sort of depends on the circumstances."

"I know what you mean," one of them chimed in. "When I want to bake bread my mother say, 'No, you too young,' and when I be bad she say, 'You old enough to know better.' "

The answer had amused me then. Now I considered it seriously. Every day the children asked me a question. "Can you walk yet?" And always with that assurance, "We prayed for you." Suddenly I was overcome with shame. I'd taken all they had to offer, but had given nothing in return. One hundred and fifty children believed I would walk.

Using all the willpower I could summon, I forced myself to slide from the bed until my feet touched the floor. Half in, half out of bed, I lay there shaking, terrified.

"God! I can't do it."

With a tremendous effort I brought my body to a sitting position with my feet planted firmly on the floor. Then I wiggled, first one hip, then the other, bringing my uncooperative body more nearly to the center of the bed.

"I will walk." With this determination I was able to slide one leg back into position on the bed, then the other. Exhausted, I fell into a deep sleep.

When Sister Amelia came with my supper that night, I asked her to help me stand. She was reluctant at first, fearing she might harm me, but when I slid from the bed, as I had done earlier in the day, and she saw I was determined, she helped me. Within the week I was walking—with halting, awkward steps, but I walked.

Father Noonan beamed when I showed him what I could do. "You are the ninth wonder of the world," he said. "I honestly never thought I'd see you walk again."

At the end of the week Father Lobsinger took me to Tofino in their boat, *The Ave*, to see the doctor. I thanked him for all he had done for me.

"Don't thank me," he said, shaking his head. "I didn't do it. Keep warm and dry now and you'll do all right."

It had been a long six weeks, but I would be all right. I knew it. It had been accomplished, surely with the doctor's help, but more especially because so many children believed God could do anything.

I felt good going back to Christie in *The Ave*. I'd completed my instruction, with the children's help, of course, and tomorrow I was to be received into the church. Rose and Alban's oldest daughter, Vera, had asked to be my patron. There was no one I would rather have had. Rose and I were close, we had been friends for a long time. It seemed right that her fourteen-year-old daughter should sponsor me.

It was evening by the time Father Lobsinger dropped the anchor of *The Ave* in the bay that fronted Christie. Christie boasted no dock. Larger boats anchored out, as in my own cove. Rowboats made the trip to shore. The only difference was that there, at Christie, mighty waves rolled in from the Pacific. You had to catch them at the right moment, then row for your life. Our moment was wrong, I realized suddenly. The surf behind us was piling up and up, with nowhere to go except into our boat. As the boat dragged on the sandy bottom, the surf overtook us, leaving us sitting in a boat full of water.

"I'll carry you to shore," Father Lobsinger said.

"Never mind," I retorted. "I'm a mite wet anyway."

A mink darting past me and into the bush brought me back to the present. I wandered back into the kitchen, all rosy pink and shiny and clean. Slim had brought me out this spring, bringing along a couple of lengths of stovepipe to replace those that would have rusted. Winter's dampness does dastardly things to pipes. He had cleaned my stove, made sure my waterline was connected, even chopped some of the wood Pat had thoughtfully provided last fall. And, of course, my boat was back in the water. Who could ask for anything more?

Chapter 48

"Hello up there!"

The shout came from the beach. I'd just emerged from the bush behind the house, where I'd been cutting a trail. I hadn't heard the whine of an engine, the trees shutting out all sounds. Now, as I recognized Bill's voice, I began to run.

"I'm coming," I yelled, dropping my clippers on the kitchen porch as I raced by it.

Bill's laughter greeted me from the beach. "One of these days," he said as I came up beside him and Joan, "going at them steps like a blamed cyclone, you're going to take off at the top and miss every damn step. I'm not sure you didn't miss a few this time." The laughter was still there, and it was contagious. Joan and I joined in.

"Doesn't look like you got slowed down much last winter," Joan observed.

"Thank heavens!" I agreed. "Oh, I'm glad to see you. Haven't seen a soul since I arrived, except for Slim, of course."

"That's what I told Bill . . . I bet you hadn't. The men are all getting ready to go fishing. Once they go, we women are stranded. Darn men . . . never satisfied to fish in their own area. Always have to be off to Kyuquot or Tofino or some darn place. Anyway, I told Bill, 'We're going now before you take off.' Oh, he gets home occasionally, but there's always something comes up . . . the waterline's broken, or the roof's leaking, or the float's sinking. Wish we lived closer so we could commiserate over a cup of tea."

I giggled. "I bet you don't spend much time commiserating. And speaking of tea, how about . . . ?"

"Uh-uh! Those steps of yours do me out. I've lost my breath before I'm halfway up. We brought tea and a lunch." She pointed to a basket sitting on the rocks. "We'll eat right here on the beach as usual, if you don't mind."

And even if I did mind, I thought to myself. Joan wasn't the only one to complain of my steps. Mrs. McLean found them difficult, too. To me they were nothing. I was used to them. Bill, with his long legs, could take them two at a time, I was sure, but Joan was small, shorter than I and more solidly built. Her home was on a flat, no steps to climb. I sympathized with her disapproval of mine. At any rate, a picnic on the beach was much to my liking. I lived in the outdoors, going inside only to sleep or to eat.

A walk in the rain could be delightful, I'd discovered. In my short shorts, if the wet brush slapped my legs it didn't matter. I walked under the trees, listening to the whispered rush of the leaves, a sound so constant it seemed no sound at all. I drank in the fragrance of the forest as I squished in the evergreen needles under my feet. I spotted spiderwebs, so heavy with droplets of rain I marveled they didn't break. I walked the beach, the rain spanking the water. *Spat! Spat! Spat!* I sloshed through my streams as they tumbled over the rocks in their rush to the sea.

"Where are you?" Joan asked.

"I'm sorry. I was thinking about how much nicer it is to be outside. I'm glad you brought a picnic lunch." I'd have to watch it, I reproved myself silently. Being alone so much, my mind tended to wander off on a course of its own. "How did you know I was back?" I asked.

Bill's laughter burst upon us, echoing back from the rocky cliffs beyond the cove. "News spreads fast in this country. Everyone knows every move you make."

"That's awful," I protested. "I like feeling I can do as I please."

"After what happened to you last winter, you'd better be glad the world cares," Joan said severely. "Though I must say, looking at you, it's hard to believe anything happened. But you are rather balmy, you know, staying here alone after an experience like that. Bill was at Queens Cove when Slim delivered the bread. When Bill came home he said, 'Well, she's back.' And I said, 'Oh, no, she *can't* be!' "

It didn't surprise me that Dr. and Mrs. McLean came out. I remembered their concern when Father Lobsinger hadn't appeared last September. In the city people seem to flow around you, but out in the bush each visit is an event, each person is someone special. They brought some of the young people from the mission with them. One young man in particular claimed my attention. He had just recently come from a farm in Alberta. Everything about the coast fascinated and intrigued him, most especially my cove and my old log house. He was full of questions. Alfred Birtles was his name. I had a feeling I'd be seeing much more of this young man.

Father Larkin came in his boat. One of the Indians had given him a salmon. He didn't say he was keeping tabs on me, but I was sure he was.

"You fix the rest of the dinner," he bade me. "I'll take care of the salmon. Can't trust a woman to prepare it the way it should be."

Dirk came in and pounded some nails. Dirk could always find something that needed fixing. This time it was my steps.

I set out for myself all the hardest jobs I could think of. I went to work on some of the large rolls of that fir Pat had cut for me, wedging them into quarters, proud I could still swing my six-pound sledgehammer without losing my breath. I cut paths to my berry patches, knowing I'd have to hack at them again before the berries ripened. I cut back the brush from the little cottage, freeing it to the sun, and I slashed my way to an old chicken coop I'd spotted high up on a bluff, almost overcome by the brush. And every day I went rowing, sometimes fishing. Muscles, not there when first I'd arrived, began to develop, along with several calluses.

It was an unpredictable April, but I had long sunny days,

and a cessation of visitors. This I'd expected. After all, they'd checked and I was okay. I watched those curious creatures, the mink, chasing each other with screams of such shrillness it set my teeth on edge. Whether they were playing or mating or fighting I couldn't determine, but whatever, my presence did nothing to deter them. One day I came upon one of them in my wild strawberry patch. There was as yet no sign of berries, but my plants were lush and green, and I wasn't quite certain I appreciated having a mink scooting among them. He *was* scooting, arching his neck, rubbing his head in the leaves, all the while emitting plaintive little mews, so unlike the screams I'd grown accustomed to.

"Are you trying to tell me something?" I asked him.

His answer was another mew, and he looked up at me with eyes that seemed to plead. I bent for a closer look. On his back, just above his tail, was a gaping hole. It looked as if some rapacious creature, maybe one of his own kind, had bitten out a good chunk of flesh. The hole was festered and flyblown, an ugly red.

"Oh, you poor thing! Somebody sure got the best of you. Don't go away now. I'll help you."

In Wally's bag there was a puffer tube of medicated powder. If I could fill the hole with the powder, it should promote some healing. I ran as fast as I could, afraid my mink might scoot off into the bushes, but when I got back he was still there, waiting, as if he'd known I'd come. I bent over for another look, then hesitated. I'd seen how, with his sharp teeth, he'd shredded the fish he caught. It had made my blood run cold until I reminded myself he'd been endowed with those teeth for just such a purpose. I could hardly condemn him for doing what was natural, and essential, if he was to live. But now I had second thoughts about those teeth. I'd have to squeeze my tube hard to get in enough powder to do any good. The rush of air and the feel of the powder could be startling in so sensitive an area. I knew how quickly he could turn about, almost doubling his body as he sprang. I stood a good chance of losing a chunk of my own flesh.

But the plea in those eyes was irresistible. I knelt beside him. "Now, you be good. I'm helping you." I hoped the sound of my voice would reassure him, so I kept talking. "Lie still as you can. This won't hurt, really it won't, and afterwards you'll feel much better."

Holding the tube directly above the wound, my heart accelerating, I squeezed hard, and powder shot from the tube, right where I wanted it to go. I held my breath, but my mink made no move. I, too, remained motionless. He could still mistake too sudden a motion on my part for a sign of attack.

"Well now, Jasper, you're a good kid."

I got to my feet. There was no move yet from my mink. The powder was soothing, containing an anesthetic which should help take some of the fire from the wound. He lay there a few minutes, as if undecided, then pushed himself up on his feet and, with one last look at me, trotted off into the bushes, leaving me to wonder why he had sought me out, what instinct had told him I could, and would, help. The mink were accustomed to my presence. They knew where I walked, but the special intelligence that had prompted him to submit to my treatment was something I couldn't explain.

A few days later, when I was out looking for shells on the low tide, I heard a soft padding behind me. I stopped and turned to look. The creature behind me had stopped, too, and met my glance.

"Is that you, Jasper?"

He made no move to run off, so I took a few steps toward him. If I could just see that tail area!

"Ah! It is you, Jasper. I'm glad you're okay."

He was okay. The wound was covered with new tissue, a healthy pink. Soon the hair would start to grow back. I felt good. My first effort alone had been a success.

I continued on around the cove, stopping and stooping whenever some shiny shell caught my eye. Jasper followed at my heels, stopping when I did, snatching up a crab or some other wiggling delicacy left stranded by the outgoing tide.

Chapter 49

I'd finished my supper and was sitting on the beach watching the sun slowly slide toward the peak of Mount Eliza. I watched a troller chugging up the inlet from the sea. It was probably headed for Zeballos, though it was rather late to be going so far. It would be dark long before they got there, not that that would stop anyone if they really wanted to go. I was puzzled, however, that the troller hugged the Nootka shoreline rather than Center Island, where there were no reefs to plague a wary seaman. I decided it was an Indian from Nuchatlitz taking the shorter route.

To my surprise, the troller did not go by, but turned and entered the cove.

"Thank heavens the tide is high," I muttered to myself. "I hope he knows where my reefs are."

He knew, for he never hesitated, coming to a stop just far enough back from the shore to avoid scraping bottom. He stuck his head out the side window, and I recognized him at once—Wilson Little, Pat's father.

"Wilson! This is a surprise. I thought you were heading for Zeballos."

"No, I come here. You can come to a party?" It was almost more demand than question. "I will take you," he added.

"A party! Oh, fun! I'll hurry and get ready."

"You okay like you are."

"Oh, but, Wilson," I objected, "if it's a party I'd like to dress up. I have a dress. I brought one. Please let me change."

"Okay. I wait."

I changed quickly, then pulled my skiff to shore and paddled out as far as the rope that secured it to shore would allow. It was far enough. Wilson gave me a hand and pulled me aboard.

"It's wonderful of you to invite me to your party," I told him on the way over.

His grunt was noncommittal, but then he asked, "You can stay all night?"

For a fraction of a second I hesitated. Certainly I hadn't come prepared to spend the night, but . . . "No reason I can't," I answered cheerfully.

Twilight softened the huddle of unpainted frame houses that was Nuchatlitz. Nuchatlitz . . . meeting place of the winds, and certainly, on that flat little island which defied the sweep of the Pacific, the winds could race in from every direction. This night was a flat calm. I was amazed by the trollers, two and three deep, lining either side of the floating dock. Even the yellow pigeon was there, in a special reserved spot. It came to me that this was a party of some importance, and I was thankful I'd insisted on changing to a dress. Wilson tied up alongside one of the trollers, and we scrambled over their decks to the dock.

"You go to Rose," he said.

Rose welcomed me with open arms and a kiss on the cheek. She always had, but now there was a subtle difference. I was almost a member of the family. Vera was my patron. Momentarily I regretted that the party couldn't have been held after school was out so Vera could be here, but as quickly realized that couldn't be, for then the trollers would all be out in the fishing grounds. I forgot all about it in the bustle going on around me. Rose finished frosting a cake almost two feet long.

"My goodness, Rose, I've never seen such a cake. Is it somebody's birthday?"

"You will see. We go now."

She led me to the community house. As she opened the door the warm smell of many bodies and the music of voices and laughter flowed out to include me. The soft glow of lamps fastened along the wall shone on the happy faces of my Indian friends, all of whom I had met at one time or another, many of whom I knew well. Father Lobsinger and Father Larkin came to greet me. I could feel myself flushing with excitement. Father Lobsinger led me to one of the benches surrounding the room. Rose had bustled off, speaking to one person and then another. They nodded, moving toward the benches, which soon were filled with mothers holding babies on their laps, little ones squeezed between father and mother. The men sat with their arms folded, their feet planted firmly on the floor.

The party was about to begin. Alban rose and walked to the center of the room. Nuchatlitz was his village and he was the chief. The party would not begin until he gave the signal. Alban was not much inclined to speech, always willing to let Rose do the talking, smiling and nodding agreement. Rather slight and not too tall, with black hair and brown skin, he was a handsome man. I was glad that, even if only because of patronage, I could claim a connection with his family. Then he began to speak, and I listened intently, not wanting to miss one word.

"We have all come together here at Nuchatlitz to honor someone we know, someone we like. She is our friend. Because of her, a great yellow bird now flies over our villages."

I was stunned, disbelieving, barely able to throttle the gasp that rose in my throat. This party was for me. I turned to Father Lobsinger.

Smiling, he shook his head. "I had nothing to do with it. This was their own idea."

The chief of each village, in turn, made his speech. The speeches were long, rambling, and highly poetic.

"Dr. Flynn was our friend. He was a good man. His wife is good woman. We are welcome in her home. She is welcome in our homes. We are friends together. Dr. Flynn had a beautiful ma-chitle [plane; the spelling is mine]. Now that beautiful ma-chitle belongs to all of us. It belongs to us because this good woman wanted us to have it. Indian people like to fly. Now Indian people can fly. Now the priests can come often to our villages."

They spoke in a soft, guttural singsong manner. The chiefs were followed by the elders, whose speeches were equally long and equally flowery. A few spoke in their own tongue. Anthony John, from Queens Cove, squeezed in beside me, translating those words I couldn't understand. It hardly would have been necessary, as the speeches carried the same theme, though each speaker vied with the others to make his speech the longest and most glowing. I wondered, a hot flush on my face, how I could possibly be as great as I was depicted. Common sense told me I wasn't. They had simply been carried away by their own rhetoric and their love of drama. Nevertheless, fact or fiction, it was uncommonly pleasant to listen to such unrestrained acclaim.

Suddenly the speeches came to an end. A hushed silence again, as all eyes focused on me. My moment of glory was over. Figuratively, the ball had been passed to me. I quivered; my stomach flip-flopped, and my knees knocked in rhythm with my heart. Slowly I unsqueezed myself from the bench and stood up. Still not a sound. Everyone waited. A smile froze on my face, my tongue stuck to the roof of my mouth, and my throat muscles were paralyzed. The first word was a croak. I swallowed hard, moistened my lips, and tried again. I could never remember my exact words, but I managed to convey my happiness at having so many good friends, my joy at being with them this night. There was no rhetoric in my speech. It was short and stumbling, but that didn't matter. The applause was thunderous.

From somewhere in the background an old phonograph ground out a popular song. Rose and Alban walked to the middle of the floor and began to dance, not an Indian dance but the white man's way. No one else moved. It puzzled me until the music stopped suddenly just as the dancing couple came to a halt directly in front of me. They separated, Alban bowing to me, Rose to Father Lobsinger. He grinned and stood up, his blue eyes twinkling. I followed his example, and as the music started again, we were whisked away in the respective arms of Alban and Rose.

Each time the music stopped, those of us on the floor bowed to someone seated until everyone there was crowded onto the floor, except for the children, who slept peacefully on the benches, unmindful of the racket. I danced and danced, wishing it never had to end. Promptly at midnight, the music stopped, and everyone returned to the benches. The children were awakened, no fussing, no crying. I sat between Father Lobsinger and Father Larkin.

"Did you dance?" I asked Father Larkin. "I didn't see you."

"I shoved them around," he said. He laughed, and I joined in. He was built to shove anyone around. His feet might not have known what he was doing, but anyone in his grasp would have been hard put not to follow whatever he did.

There was no time for more comments. A couple of the men carried in a table covered with a gleaming white tablecloth and set it in front of us. A procession of women followed with an array of sweets it would be hard to equal . . . lemon pies, berry pies, chocolate cakes, white cakes, plates of cookies. There was Freshie, similar to Kool-Aid, for the children, and pots and pots of coffee for the adults. I had to taste a little of everything.

"So good!" I murmured over and over.

And always, with a shy smile, "I made it."

I noticed the crowd had thinned, and I supposed they had gone off to sleep, in their houses, on their boats, wherever. I was wrong. They reappeared now in costume. Colorful replicas of the whale were stitched on the men's white shirts. There were black and purple bands around the bottoms of the white overblouses worn by the women. There was a red band over the right shoulder and a blue band over the left. They met in a V over the chest and were secured with a white ribbon bow. The small hats they wore were also decorated with ribbons. Some clutched what looked like miniature harpoons. Others wielded what I took to be paddles. Then, to the beat of the drum and the rhythmic chant of the participants, the dancing began. I had never before witnessed such a dance, but I felt certain it had to do with their whaling expeditions of earlier years. I knew of their reputation as the greatest whalers of all time.

The room shook to the pounding of their feet; the lamps swung. Hands clapped in unison, and I found myself joining in the chant, a chant led by the drummer as he thumped with his hands on a drum made of deerhide, soaked and scraped and beaten until it was soft and stretchable, then mellowed by many years.

They danced their way from the room, but the show was not over. Sophie appeared wearing a colorful wooden head-dress of the eagle. Her dress was concealed by a black shawl with fringe extending to the hem of her dress. Sophie was one of the oldest women there, surely in her seventies, but she could dance and she knew it. She looked proud and beautiful as she stomped and twirled to the beat of the drum.

There were more dances, dances with knives, dances with arrows, and after the dancing there were games, running, jumping games, and I joined in, laughing with them over my mistakes and miscalculations. I forgot I'd ever once thought of sleep.

It was well past three in the morning. Mothers slipped away, carrying sleeping children in their arms. Older children clung to their fathers, clutching his pants leg, his shirt, what-ever came to hand.

"Come," Rose said. "Your bed is ready."

Hand in hand, we walked through the darkened village to her house. Without my hand in hers I would have stumbled and fallen. She knew every hole, every hump in the uneven ground.

Chapter 50

"Slim! You of all people! I never ever thought you'd scrape bottom."

"Shallowed out sooner than I thought," Slim admitted. "Well, I can't think of a nicer place to be stranded. Hand me your rope. I'll tie your skiff alongside. You can hop aboard and share my lunch while we wait for the tide to give me a boost."

"I could make lunch, if you'd like to come up to the house," I offered.

"Thank you, but I'd better stick with the *Lady*. Never can tell what the tide might do. Could swing me up against one of your reefs. Don't worry about food. I carry plenty, and if I should run out," he added with a chuckle, "your whole box of groceries is sitting right here."

I scrambled up over the side of the *Misty Lady* and sat on a bench while Slim made coffee and got out the sandwiches he'd made before he left home. He had all sorts of goodies besides—oranges, carrots, and celery sticks.

"I like to chaw on them as I go along," he said. "Maybe you'd like to peek at your mail while you're sitting there. Might be something important."

There were the usual letters . . . one from Maureen, one from Mama, and one from my sister, Berne, as well as letters from friends. Nothing really urgent, I decided. I could read them later. As I went to tuck them back in my grocery box, my hand rested on Berne's letter. Awfully flat! She generally wrote pages. Puzzled, I ripped it open, my eyes scanning the single sheet.

"My gosh!" I exclaimed. "My sister and her husband are coming up from Los Angeles to visit me for a week, the first of July, she says. What's the date today, Slim?"

"Oh, seventeenth or eighteenth of June, somewhere around there."

"I'll have to buy a lot more food. I'd better start making a list. I don't know what accommodations Berne and Jack are expecting, but can you bring them out, Slim?"

"Why not?" His answer was casual, but his grin was broad. Slim wouldn't have it any other way, I suspected. He knew everybody in the country, knew everyone's comings and goings. He'd not want to miss out on Berne and Jack.

For the first time since I'd arrived, I started counting the days. Berne was checking on me, no doubt. She'd not thought I was too bright, returning to the wilds so soon after my paralysis. Whatever, I was glad they were coming.

The day dawned bright and beautiful, as if it knew that for city dwellers it had to present its very best face. I was up and down my steps a dozen times, anticipating their arrival, hoping to catch a first glimpse of the *Misty Lady* as she rounded the northern tip of Center Island, finally deciding I might just as well stay on the beach.

When the *Misty Lady* did round the bend, my first inclination was to get into my skiff and row out, which would have been foolish, for it would take the *Lady* at least twenty minutes to reach my islands. Finally, I could stand it no longer. I got into the skiff and paddled around the cove, waiting impatiently for Slim to skirt my reefs.

"Berne! Jack!"

"That's enough of a load," he said. "Come back for their bags and your groceries."

I rowed them to shore, then rowed back to the *Misty Lady*.

"You're a fine one," Slim scolded me with a roguish grin. "Why didn't you tell me you two don't look any more like sisters than I look like Alban? Almost missed them. I was looking for a blond mite like yourself. Then this tall brunette hops off the *Uchuck*, five ten if she's an inch. 'There's another one George kept on board for the night,' I said to myself. But then a man followed her and no one else got off, so I figured I'd better ask. It was them, all right."

I grinned back at him. "I'm so used to us being different, I never once gave it a thought, Slim."

"Maybe you'd best give them a thought now. They look kind of lost standing there on the beach by themselves."

"Okay, Slim. See you next week, rain or shine. They have to get back even if the sky falls." With a shove off from the *Misty Lady* and a wave of the hand, I left him.

"You wrote about it, but I still can't believe it," Berne said as I pulled up to the shore. "Two hours on Slim's boat and we didn't pass one single house. Now he's gone and here we are, surrounded by nothing."

"Surrounded by everything, you mean," I corrected her. "Oh, not houses, like you're used to, but . . ." I paused helplessly, my hands outstretched. How did one describe what surrounded me here?

"It's beautiful, all right," Berne agreed. "In fact, I've never seen a more beautiful place."

"And too beautiful a day to waste," Jack broke in. "If you girls don't mind, I'll carry this stuff up to the house. Then I'm going to change my clothes and go fishing. I can borrow your skiff and your rod?"

"Absolutely! Would you like me to go along, just for a little while, to show you how?"

For a moment there was dead silence, then two words: "I've fished." They said all I needed to know.

Berne got herself settled and then changed her clothes so I could show her around. Remembering back to our school years, when I'd had to almost run to keep up with her long legs, I set out at a brisk pace back through the trees, following trails I'd hacked out, around the beach to the cottage, and up the bluff behind it.

"It's fantastic," she admitted, "but so alone! Why do you always have to go to such extremes?"

I shrugged. There was no logical answer. What makes one person seek the cities while another can't get far enough away? Something deep inside, I reckoned, a built-in antenna that directs you in the direction you're to go, something I couldn't quite put into words.

Berne had sunk down on the steps. "I'm beat," she said. "Do you know how much I walk at home? From the house to the car, from the car to the office. That's it. I had no idea what I was getting into here. Just around the cove to the cottage, you said. Sounded like nothing. I'll bet it's a good two city blocks, and rocks to stumble over every foot of the way."

"You'll get used to it," I assured her. "When you get rested a bit maybe we can mosey on out to the inlet and see how Jack's making out. It's easier going, a nice mossy path through the trees." I grinned at her. "Part of your trouble is that your shoes are all wrong. Those open-toed thongs might be all right for a sandy beach, but on my rocks . . ." I shook my head disapprovingly.

"You're telling me! I think I've worn a blister between my toes, too."

"Gosh! I'm sorry. Why didn't you say something?"

"Pride! Couldn't admit even to myself I'd gone soft. I brought some tennis shoes. I'll put them on next time."

"Can you make it back to the house now?"

"I can, because I'm starving. All this exertion, combined with your air. I feel like I haven't eaten in days. It's time we started dinner anyway, isn't it?"

We started dinner much earlier than I ever had. But fresh air and exercise do make you hungry, I admitted, especially when you've just come from a big smoggy city and your lungs and your body aren't adjusted to the invigorating effect of clean air. Berne assured me I didn't need to worry about meat. Jack would undoubtedly bring in a fish, or two, or three. I said nothing, but I laid out the steaks I'd had Slim bring out.

"Must have been the wrong time of the day to catch fish," Jack observed later, absolving himself. "I'll get up early in the morning and go out."

He did, early, and so quietly that I didn't even know he'd left. He came in about noon, tired and hungry, with no fish. Moreover, he'd sunburned his ankles. And in getting in and out of the skiff he'd gotten his tennis shoes and the cuffs of his pants wet. They were sun-dried, encrusted with salt and irritating to skin not used to exposure. I suggested we wash both pants and shoes.

"These pants are all right," he objected. "I really don't want to put on another pair. This is no place for good pants."

"I've got an old pair of Wally's you can wear. They'll fit you short, but that's good. They won't be dangling around your sore ankles."

He agreed, though a trifle reluctantly, and Berne took them outside to shake them in case they'd collected dust in the couple of years they'd been hanging around. Her yell startled me.

"Bethine!"

I ran. Maybe a snake had slithered over her foot. That could be disconcerting if you weren't prepared. Or maybe a little mouse had scurried through the grass. They were always with me, inside and out. I'd prepared Berne and Jack for that, if indeed you can prepare anyone. At least, I'd tried.

"What's the matter?" I demanded, rushing up to her.

"Look!" She pointed to the ground. "I shook it out of Wally's pants."

I stared, incredulous, then dropped to my knees. Berne was beside me, helping me to gather up the green paper money that had floated from Wally's pants pocket.

"Wonder how much there is," Berne speculated.

"I don't know. How much have you got?"

"Better count it."

So we sat there on the ground, counting our loot—just over one hundred dollars. When she spoke, Berne's voice sounded strange, almost strangled.

"How come you never looked in his pockets?"

"I don't know. I never looked in them when he was alive. Why should I look in them when he's dead?"

She knelt there, shaking her head. "Sometimes I don't know about you. What are you going to do with your windfall, anyway?"

"Well, first of all, I'll get me a hot fudge sundae. I really get a craving for ice cream sometimes, even dream about it."

"Okay, but that isn't going to cost you a hundred dollars."

"Oh, I've plenty of use for it, don't worry. I'll buy some shoes, something really stylish that I wouldn't wear up here. When I leave here at the end of the summer my shoes are so tattered I toss them out, except for one pair to get me back to Seattle. I'll have a ball spending that money."

I asked Jack, "How would you like to fish for trout at Owasitsa Lake tomorrow?"

"Sounds all right," he agreed. "Interesting name, anyway. Any special meaning attached to it?"

"Uh-huh! Owasitsa is Indian for 'spawning ground of the sockeye.'"

"Sounds encouraging. How is the fishing?"

"Well . . . sometimes you catch them, sometimes you don't."

Jack snorted, then grinned. "That has a familiar ring. At any rate, I can't do any worse than I have up to now. How far is it?"

"Not far. We can take the skiff to the river, about a quarter of a mile from here. Then it's about a seven-eighths-of-a-mile hike back through the trees. It's a beautiful lake."

"Let's hope the fishing is beautiful. You want to come, Berne?"

"You'd better believe it. I'm not going to be left here alone."

We set out the next morning in high spirits. Jack rowed us to the mouth of the river, and we tied our skiff to a limb protruding out over the water. It was easy going at first, a sandbank back from the salt, then a marshy area where purple clover grew thick and tall, reaching to our knees. It was sunny and warm, and the clover matting under our feet perfumed the air. Bees rose at our approach, but their buzz was not angry and they ignored us, seeking other clover. Then we entered the forest, where spruce and hemlock, cedar and fir were crowded together, reaching up to the sky, shutting out the sun and its warmth. The air became heavy with the mingled odors of evergreens and the dank earth. I forged ahead, around stumps, under or over fallen trees, depending on how high off the ground they lay. I scrounged through bushes, sometimes floundering, down on my knees. Burdened with fishing gear and lunch sacks, it wasn't easy going.

"Hold it!" Jack called after a time. He'd fallen behind, helping Berne. "I thought you said there was a trail."

"I did."

"Well, I don't see it."

"It's just sort of grown over a bit."

"Grown over! That's what you call it. Now be honest. Are you sure you know where you are?"

"Yeah. I'm sure."

Actually I wasn't sure, but I wasn't lost, even though the trail had completely eluded me. Looking way up ahead, I could see sky, and where I saw sky there had to be lake. I pointed in that direction. My deduction elicited a skeptical shake of the head from Jack and a half smile from Berne, but they followed along. It took us two hours, but we came out where I knew we would, on a grassy area where the river flowed from the lake. We flung ourselves down on the grass, humping our shoulders, arching and twisting our necks to relieve aching muscles.

"Let's eat," Berne suggested. "I'm glad you insisted we bring a lunch, even though it was the very devil packing it along your trail."

Jack fished after we'd eaten, casting from the shore. Berne refused to move, resting up, she insisted, for the trek back to the salt. She didn't rest too long. Jack struck out again. If he couldn't catch fish, he saw no reason to linger.

Berne groaned. "Do we have to? I'd rather swim back than tackle that trail of yours again."

"That's an idea," Jack agreed. "I don't fancy following you along another trail, either. How about following the river back?"

"No good! The brush is so thick along the river at this point we could never fight our way through it." I paused, considering. "The brush does thin out down a ways, and the river's only deep here, where it joins the lake. We could head back through the trees for a short way, then cut back to the river and wade out to the salt. There'll be rocks. . . ." I looked at Berne.

"Give me the rocks. I'm all for the river."

It was as I had said, rocky and slippery but shallow. The sun filtered through the tops of the trees that embraced in the sky, forming an arch over the river and letting in just enough warmth. It took us half an hour to wade out. Berne timed us, gleefully.

Jack seemed unusually thoughtful rowing home. I felt bad for him. He'd come hoping to catch fish. So far it was a lost cause. As we entered the channel into the cove, he broke the silence.

"I'm tired of wasting time." And he grinned. "How about showing me how to fish?"

"Hey! I'd love to. We'll dump that trout line up at the house, pick up the other pole, and be on our way. Want to come, Berne?"

"No thank you. I'm for a nap. But don't you be gone over half an hour."

I showed Jack how I let the line slip slowly to the bottom, lifting it up and down with quick little jerks. In no time I had a snapper.

"That simple!" Jack groaned. "If I hadn't been so disgustingly smart we could have had fish every meal."

"You can still get all you can eat. Row me back in, then stay out as long as you like."

It rained the next two days, but that didn't keep Jack in. He fished every day until Slim came again, and we ate fish at every meal except breakfast. If ever a man was happy! The day that they had to leave came just too fast.

"I'm sorry it rained," I apologized as they boarded Slim's boat.

"Don't apologize," Berne protested. "We'd have felt cheated if we hadn't experienced your rain. It's been a fabulous vacation, and I think, after seeing you in action, I can stop worrying about you. But you write every week, hear?"

As I climbed the bluff back to the house, my world seemed extraordinarily quiet. I paused and looked around. Even a mouse stirring in the bush would be a welcome sound. No mouse, no mink, not even the chirp of a bird! Where were all my friends? Then I heard a rustle in the bushes, and Minniebelle appeared, strutting audaciously along the path.

Chapter 51

Not too many visitors appeared after Berne and Jack left. The weather was right for fishing, and fishermen would be out for the catch. My most frequent visitor was Father Larkin, and he often never even got out of his boat.

"Hallow!" he'd bellow from the cove. "Everybody okay up there?"

"Everybody," of course, was me. Rather a nice designation. It amused me.

I'd been hearing many boats these last weeks, but seldom bothered to run down. Too many boats, this time of the year, just passing by. More people from Tahsis, mill workers mainly, had gotten speedboats. Since people were bound to go, and there were no roads, speedboats had replaced cars in the affections of the populace. When the men weren't working, they were roaring up and down the inlets. Where didn't matter. Also, a logging outfit had gone in up Espinosa Inlet, too far away for me to witness their activities, but close enough that I could see the ugly scar on the side of a once green mountain. I avoided looking in that direction. The scar provoked a like scar in my heart, a wound that would take as long to heal as it took the mountainside to recoup. I recognized that logging was indispensable to the area, but I wished it could have been farther away from my door. Out of sight, out of mind, so to speak.

The loggers, too, at the end of the day would join the noisy parade that disturbed the tranquility of my inlet. Oh, yes, it *was* mine. All those others were trespassers to whom noise and confusion was a way of life. How could they appreciate the quiet beauty of the area when the noise of their engines blocked out the cries of the gulls and the smell of the gas they burned polluted the atmosphere? Sure, they were far enough from my shores that I couldn't smell the gas, but I knew the smell was there and I was disturbed. I gloated over those days when there were no boats in the inlet, and there were many, for men must work. Most of the invasion was confined to the weekends. Then I would seek the back trails where the trees blocked out the sounds on the inlet.

Not all sounds were unwanted. I knew the whine of Father Larkin's boat when it was turning into the cove. I ran down when I heard it this morning.

"Time for a coffee?" I asked as I leaped from the bottom step to a landing on the beach.

"None! Not this time. Got a wedding this afternoon. Need a little time to get out of these clothes and into something more priestly."

"Next time then, Father."

"It's a deal."

It was the same story each time with Father Lobsinger. Whenever I heard that familiar drone in the skies, I would run to see the old yellow pigeon. Sometimes she came close, dipping a wing in passing, and I stood there on the beach, a lump in my throat, remembering old times. The Indian people felt now that that plane was their own private passport. There were many needs.

"My mother's sick down at Ahousat. I got to see her. You take me, Father?"

Some cases were urgent . . . a little girl badly burned, rushed to a hospital.

For me it was enough to know that the pigeon was up there, doing her job.

Though I didn't have many visitors those hot July weeks, I

had the home folks: Minniebelle the grouse mother, Tessie and Jasper, my friendly mink, and of course Reuben and Rachel, my noisy gulls, who invited their friends. Oscar, the seal, made the cove his headquarters. That silly face, that always looked like it was grinning, could brighten even a dull day. There were the jays and the squirrels, quarreling over my filberts, not pets especially, for the only things with which I could entice them, those still-green filberts, they were more adept at gathering than I, but I loved their chatter and their games. Though they didn't seek me out, neither did they shun me. I was a part of their world, a fixture. To the crows, also, I suspected, I was hardly more than a fixture. In their search for clams and other delights from the sea, they'd hop a step or two, just enough to get out of my way, a saucy *caw, caw* suggesting I'd intruded.

The mink had taken over my beach. One, I knew, had to be Jasper, for he still dogged my footsteps. Another I had called Tessie. I wasn't certain she was female, of course, but a certain gentleness suggested it. She was smaller than Jasper, more delicate in appearance. She hung around the beach, alert for any perch that ventured into the cove. Into the water! Was any creature more swift? Then she'd emerge, her brown body sleek and shining, and always a fish clutched between those two rows of fearsome white teeth. Often she'd lay it on the rocks at my feet. An offering? Never offended that I rejected her gift, she'd pick it up and trot off into the bushes.

One hot day I went to the outside beach and sat hunched on a boulder, staring out over the inlet. So quiet, I thought. Nice! And then, somewhere behind me, I heard a series of sharp little squeals. Jasper? Or was it Tessie? As I turned to look, my eyes widened in astonishment. It was Tessie. No doubt now that she was female. Behind her trailed five little mink. She paused, craning her neck, as she studied me. The five remained motionless, awaiting her decision. Then it began again, those peculiar high-pitched cries. I knew what she was saying.

"It's okay, kids. It's only Mrs. Flynn."

She trotted over the rocks behind me, and the kids followed along, single file, all talking at once. With remarkable agility Tessie scrambled up a cliff, stopping at the top to mark the progress of her youngsters. They tried and fell back. She scolded, and they tried again, but their legs were too short, their coordination undeveloped. Even as I wondered how she would overcome this obstacle, she anchored the sharp nails of her hind feet into a crevice in the cliff, slung her body over the cliff, and held out a paw to a struggling child. The child took the offered paw and was pulled up the cliff. In like manner all five reached the top of the cliff.

"Tessie," I said to myself, "how long have you had those kids hidden back there in the bushes? No wonder you spent so much time fishing." And I wondered, as I looked at the cliff where they had scrambled up and beyond my line of vision, if maybe Jasper was the father of those kids, if maybe he had sustained that bite fighting another male for Tessie's favors.

When Tessie had interrupted me I'd been watching sockeye jumping in the inlet as they made their way to their spawning grounds at Owasitsa Lake.

"Too bad the Fisheries has posted my area off limits," I'd told Bill one time.

"Not at all," he'd replied. "The salmon have to be protected. Anyway, they're not biting when they're jumping."

But the area was not off limits to the gulls. There'd be all those dead bodies lying around after the salmon had spawned, and maybe even a few succulent eggs that floated away before they could be properly buried. Sockeye bury their spawn up to eighteen inches deep, Bill said, butting the gravel aside with their heads and their bodies, a herculean task that left them battered and broken. I marveled at the incredible compulsion involved in the spawning process.

With so many predators lying in wait, it was a miracle so many salmon reached their spawning ground.

There was one predator I wanted to see in action, even though Bill had warned me against it. "Keep away from the black bear when they're fishing," he'd said. "Generally they won't bother you, unless they feel threatened, but when they're catching fish they're ornerier than hell."

Maybe, but I still wanted to see. And what better time than now? The waters in the inlet were fairly quiet. I could row to the mouth of Owasitsa River and watch from there. Bill need never know. Still, I approached the river cautiously, dipping my paddles silently and keeping well out from the shore. Contrarily, doing something I'd been cautioned against gave me a pleasant tingly feeling, sort of like taking a dare. I caught my breath: There was a bear. I was in luck. He didn't look frightening, but quite powerful. As I watched, he scooped up a sockeye. Then, the head in his mouth, the tail dangling, he ambled off into the bushes. I should have been satisfied, but I sat as if anchored to the spot with an unseen line, and I watched, entranced, as my bear repeated the process over again.

"You'd never believe," Bill had said, "how fast those beasts can move."

I could neither outrun nor outrow him, but I stayed on until he disappeared into the bush and didn't return. I turned then, still dipping my oars silently as I moved out and away from the river. Not until I was in the deeper waters of the inlet, with my skiff bucking the gentle chop of the waves, did I really bend to the oars, exerting all the energy I could muster.

That evening, as I carried my garbage out to dispose of it, I heard voices, faintly, floating to me from away off over the water. Curious, I ran to the tree line, where I could look out over the inlet, seeing without being seen. It was a balmy evening. Not even a whisper of the wind disturbed the waters of the inlet. It was the kind of atmosphere in which sounds are intensified. Though the boat I'd spotted was a good half mile away, the voices rising above the whine of the engine were clear and defined. Not Indians! The range of their voices was too extreme, their laughter too rollicking. Loggers, probably, from up Espinosa Inlet, heading for the cove.

"Drunk!"

It was not just the erratic course of the boat that led to my conclusion. Slurred, fatuous words, laughter as silly as that from a couple of wrestling schoolboys, was all the evidence I needed. I looked down at my short shorts, hardly an appropriate costume for entertaining guests in the condition I perceived these to be in. Running back to the house, I slipped out of my shorts and into a pair of knee-highs, the most modest apparel I possessed. Not that I expected trouble, but there was no excuse for inviting it. As I changed, their voices affronted the stillness of my room. Already my guests were entering the cove.

"Maybe they'll hang up on a reef and drown," I thought wickedly as I tore down the steps to the beach. It was best, I thought, to meet them there. Maybe I could persuade them to go on their way.

They had cleared the reefs and now pulled up onto the beach with a flourish, unmindful of rocks scraping the bottom of their boat.

"You should be careful," I cautioned them. "You could dig a hole in your boat."

"Nah!" The two of them grinned up at me. "We do it all the time. This old clinker's tough built."

"Maybe," I agreed, "but even a little leak would be no fun. There's a lot of water between you and your camp."

"Aah! Don't worry. It ain't hurt. 'Sides, we ain't goin' nowheres, not right now anyways." And I knew that, for the moment at least, my chances of persuading them to leave were slight.

While we'd been talking, my eyes and my nose had been busy. The two cases of beer in the bottom of the boat, one pretty well disposed of, were not the only evidence they were drunk. They smelled like uncapped bottles of beer, and they weaved on unsteady feet as they stood there in their boat, reminding me of the sea grasses at the bottom of the cove that swayed with the movement of the sea. Short-sleeved knit shirts revealed muscular arms and, clinging damply to their bodies, suggested equally muscular chests. I would have known they were loggers even without the double-bitted axes lying in the boat, their blades gleaming wickedly as the lowering beams of the sun flickered upon them.

"Bet you came to give me a hand." It was a tenuous assumption.

"Yeah! Yeah, we did," the taller one answered, almost as if he'd forgotten the purpose of their visit and thanked me for reminding him.

"Well, I do have several small mountain ash that are crowding in on my evergreens. Those axes look like they'd do the job."

I pointed out the trees, and the men went to work. They swung their axes with a rhythm that was sheer magic, first one side of the bit, then a quick toss to the other side. Masters! I had to admire them. Zing! Zing! Zing! Thud! A knot. Then zing again. Crash! Two trees down and two more to go. Drunk for sure, those two, but it had no effect on their ability to chop down trees.

Their efforts produced a more beery odor in the sweat that seemed to ooze from their bodies. Offensive in a way, but I wanted to grin. Knocking a few trees down should take some of the fire out of my unwanted guests. I doubted they had really come to chop down trees. They couldn't have known I wanted any cut down. Actually, I hadn't known it myself until I saw the axes. Anything, I had thought, to work off some of that beer and then, hopefully, send them on their way.

"Where do you want them?" one demanded as they flung their axes aside. He was the older of the two and seemed to do all the talking. Neither, I decided, could be more than thirty.

"Drag them down on the beach. When the branches dry I'll break them up for kindling."

That proved not to be too much of a job either. These men were speedy and steady on their feet now. The work had had a sobering effect.

"A good job," I said when they were finished. "Now I'll be able to look down on the water right from the house. Those trees kind of had me closed in."

"Yeah! Much better."

The younger man still remained silent, merely nodding his tousled curly head in agreement with his partner, who now strode toward the boat. "Good!" I thought. "They're leaving." The sun had dipped over Mount Eliza and evening shadows were lengthening. If they were to be back at camp before dark, there was no time for loitering. But my guests didn't concur. The big fellow reached for the full case of beer.

"Calls for a drink," he said. "We'll just haul this up to the house."

"Sorry!" My voice was firm. "Just leave that in your boat, please. I don't allow drinking here."

Two pairs of eyes regarded me in astonishment. "You've got to be kidding."

"No, I'm not kidding. Besides, if you want to get back to camp before dark . . ."

"Who said we wanted to? We know the way. Anyways, we got a light. Right now we're damned thirsty." And he reached again for the case of beer.

"Leave it there!" I hoped my voice sounded menacing. Certainly it was the only menacing thing about me. Compared to them, I reflected, I must look like a peanut. Peanut or not, no men were going to push me around, even men nice enough to cut down my encroaching trees. "If you'd like to come up to the house," I said, trying to sound more hospitable, "I'll make you some coffee and then you can be on your way."

"Coffee!" There were mutterings and grumblings, but both men followed me up the steps, leaving the case of beer lying untouched in the bottom of the boat.

My fire had died down. With all the distraction, I'd forgotten it. It took a while now to get it hot enough to set coffee to perking. I waited nervously, my eyes on the window, concerned that the night was fast overtaking my visitors. There wasn't much conversation. They'd had plenty to say out there on the water, but now they merely watched me, their heads tipping to one side, then the other, their lips pursed in a half smile that was part derision, and now and again I caught a glimmer of mischief in their eyes as covert glances passed between them. Rascals, I decided, but I ignored the glimmer, more concerned with the approaching night.

"My, it's getting dark," I said, by way of saying something. "Guess we'd best light a lamp. Sorry to keep you guys waiting so long, but the coffee's about ready now. You must be getting anxious to get started back."

"No sweat!" my talker assured me noncommittally.

The coffee was ready. I poured it and sat down facing them, fumbling for something to say. Wrapping their mugs in powerful hands, they slurped the hot brown liquid as if, in all the world, there was no other concern.

Something made me look up, and I caught, full force, the look that passed between them. That mischief in their eyes was no longer just a glimmer. It sparkled and danced, culminating in grins it would be hard to mistake.

The talker cleared his throat peremptorily. "We got a real good idea how to scare you," he said slyly, the mischief in his eyes seeming to pop out at me.

For a moment I said nothing, recalling a conversation I'd had with Father Larkin on one of his visits.

"Don't ever be afraid," he'd said. "No matter what, don't be afraid."

At the time, somewhat scornfully, I'd brushed the advice aside. Whatever in the world was there to be afraid of? But now, with those two grinning loggers sitting across from me, Father Larkin's meaning became clear.

Don't ever be afraid!

I looked into the eyes of the man who had spoken. I smiled and said pleasantly, but speaking slowly and with emphasis, "I'm sure you have, but if you do, I'll have to go back to Seattle, and I don't want to go back to Seattle. I want to live here."

For a long moment we sat, staring at each other. His eyes dropped first. "I'm sorry," he said, looking down at his shoes. "We don't aim to drive you away. You belong here."

"Thank you," I said.

Tensions and uncertainties disappeared as if a slate had

been wiped clean. Words flowed freely now, even the younger, curly-headed fellow offering a few opinions.

"I've only had a third-grade education," the older man told me, "but I have dreams and ambitions, same as any other man. I want to make something of myself, but with so little schooling I've felt I hadn't a damn chance. I've jumped from one camp to another, in trouble and out. The stories I could tell, but who wants to listen? We're all the same, in for the money, makin' a stake, then goin' for broke and right back in the old drag again."

I nodded sympathetically, then turned as the curly-haired fellow shuffled his feet.

"Could I use your washroom?" he asked formally.

"Certainly. There's a path along that row of filbert trees. Just follow it along. Better take a flashlight," I added as an afterthought. "It has really gotten dark."

"Thank you," he said, and he took the flashlight and disappeared into the night.

The other fellow had gotten to his feet, too, and had set his empty cup on the table.

My visitors noted the lateness of the hour, nearly eleven o'clock, and decided they'd best head back to camp before someone got some tomfool notion they'd drowned and set out to search. But as their voices floated back to me from over the water I knew the camp would soon be cognizant that two missing loggers were alive and in fine fettle.

And then I grinned, even giggled aloud. If it was true, as Bill had said, that everyone in the country knew my every move, tonight's episode would not go untold. The word would pass from camp to camp. "Mrs. Flynn's not one to be pushed around." I knew I had nothing more to fear from the loggers.

Chapter 52

The shrill blast of a whistle shattered the morning stillness. The *Uchuck!* Must be making the haul out to Ferrier Point again, a little later than last summer, I reflected, for here it was almost the end of July. This time Mama would not be on board, but by the sound of that whistle I'd be going along for the ride anyway. The thought put wings to my feet as I sped down the steps and climbed into my skiff.

It was the same as before—shouts and laughter and eager voices. Oh, I loved that big old boat, and I loved the crew. What other boat in the whole world the size of the *Uchuck*, I wondered, would stop in the middle of nowhere and wait for one lone woman to row out, just to go along for a ride?

I wandered around, greeting one and another, so many I knew. Then a voice, hesitant, almost shy, caught my attention.

"Mrs. Flynn?" It was a question, as if he questioned his right to address me.

"Alfred Birtles!" I exclaimed. I could hardly forget this young man from the prairies of Alberta who had come with the McLeans to visit me, who had been so delighted with my cove and my old log house. "It's good to see you. I'd hoped you would visit the cove again."

A slight pink flushed his cheeks. "That's sort of what I wanted to talk to you about, Mrs. Flynn. I'm getting married . . . to Cathy here." He reached out and took the hand of a pretty dark-haired girl.

"How wonderful. Have you set a date?"

"Yes . . . August ninth, and we want you to come. Dr. McLean said he'd send a boat out for you." Alfred gulped as he finished. The pink in his cheeks had deepened.

"I wouldn't miss it," I told them.

The conversation should have been concluded then, but Alfred shifted uneasily from one foot to the other, and an expression in Cathy's eyes told me something more was coming.

"Mrs. Flynn." He gulped again, then blurted the words out fast, as if he must say them before his courage ran out. "Mrs. Flynn, we think there's no more beautiful place in the world than your cove. Could we have our honeymoon at your place?" His face was now a deep red. I'd feared he'd choke on those last words, but they were said, and I saw his relief.

I reached out and took a hand of each of those earnest young people. "Anyone who agrees so completely with me about the beauty of my cove is more than welcome. I'll be counting the days."

"There's just one more thing, Mrs Flynn." Alfred was grinning now, suddenly brave. "You see, when you get married other people sort of try to mess things up for you. Just as a joke," he assured me quickly, as if nothing like that had ever happened to me, or if it had, I was too old to remember. "They told us we could have a boat to come out in, but we figure they'll mess with the engine and fix it so it won't run, so we decided, if it's okay with you, we'd row out after the wedding. Would you be game to row back with us?" It was a long speech for Alfred. He paused, out of breath, waiting for my reaction.

His speech quite took my breath away. The very farthest I'd rowed was to the river and back, a quarter of a mile each way. What he proposed to row was thirteen miles, more or less, depending on whether the tide was high and we could cut through the obstructing reefs or whether it was low and we had to go around them, depending also on whether we followed the shoreline or braved the choppy waters down the center of the inlet. Following the shoreline would be the longer way, of course, but it could be faster if the sea was running heavy and the wind and the tide were against us. In my mind, thirteen miles loomed like a hundred.

"Have you had a chance to do much rowing since you came to Esperanza?" I hedged.

"Some, and I'm strong as an ox. Cathy's rowed lots. She's good. We could do it easy."

"I hope you're good, because I'm not, but if you think you can do it . . . okay, I'm game." I crossed my fingers behind my back, telling myself I couldn't put the ax to so much exuberance.

Events seldom happen exactly as planned, and certainly not in an area as unpredictable as the west coast of Vancouver Island. The weather was flawless. Indeed, everyone gathered at Esperanza agreed it was a day just made for a wedding. Alfred's mother and his younger brother, Dave, had come from Alberta. Cathy's parents and the officiating minister came from Vancouver. Frank and Sophie Savey came from Nuchatlitz. There were even uninvited guests. A small cruiser, with a man and wife aboard, had come up coast from Seattle and stopped at Esperanza for gas. When an invitation was extended to them, they accepted with wholehearted enthusiasm.

Though Esperanza was a mission settlement, it boasted no church, adhering to the shantyman precept of carrying the gospel from shanty to shanty, rather than expecting the dwellers to come to a church. And in this way, I'm sure, the gospel reached a greater number of people, for loggers, fishermen, and the like are not noted churchgoers. Esperanza families held their own services in the hospital waiting room, which was large enough to accommodate their numbers. Holding services here served a dual purpose. The doors to the patients' rooms were left open, so they were included in the service whether they were so inclined or not.

A hospital waiting room, however, was hardly a place for such a joyous affair as a wedding, so it was decided it would be held out-of-doors. Butterflies flitted along the flower-embroidered lawn, and the blue waters of the inlet sparkled in the background. A more beautiful setting couldn't have been devised. The men had fashioned an altar, which the women draped with white linen and adorned with bouquets of roses which rivaled the beauty of the roses Wally and I had set out at the cove. Long tables, also draped with white linens, were set out under the evergreens for the feasting that would follow the ceremony. It all looked very proper and very festive, but Cathy insisted on one further feature. She wanted an archway that would resemble the portals of a church, and so it was fashioned and twined with roses.

The women of Esperanza bustled about with last-minute preparations for the feast, the placing of silver and glasses, the necessary condiments. Guests milled about, exchanging greetings, and about it all there was an air of expectancy. I had a glimpse of Alfred talking to the couple who had come in on the cruiser. I saw him grin, and wondered what he was up to. Then I forgot about it. Word was being passed around that the ceremony was about to begin.

Chairs had been placed so there was an aisle leading up to the altar. As we settled ourselves in our chairs, the minister took his place at the altar and was joined by Alfred and his best man. He is so handsome, I thought, and so serious in his dedication to a life in the mission field.

There was a hushed silence as the wedding march, played on a small portable organ, sent its stirring notes out over the gathering. They flowed to the mountains across the waters and echoed back, an accompaniment to an accompaniment. All heads turned as Cathy, replete with flowing veil and ankle-length layered gown, appeared on the arm of her father, slow precise steps, under the archway of roses, up the aisle between the rows of chairs. There was a flush on her cheeks and a glow of happiness that was reflected, not only in her eyes, but in her carriage, and in Alfred's eyes I saw her loveliness reflected again.

The ceremony proceeded solemnly until a sudden puff of

wind lifted Cathy's skirts and a bumblebee, confused by the swirling garments, flew into an inner fold. A murmur ran through the crowd as the distracted buzzing of the bee gathered momentum. No one moved. We sat glued to our chairs, as if the bee and its buzzing had accomplished mass hypnosis. Alfred looked helpless. Cathy's eyes were fixed, staring at nothing, but she stood stock-still. Then Cathy's mother ran forward and dropped to her knees, breaking the spell. Assisted by Cathy's attendants, she gently lifted the skirts until, among the folds, the imprisoned bee was exposed. For a moment, it clung to the fold; then, sensing it was free, it soared up and away.

Cathy smiled. Alfred grinned, and a subdued titter, like a whisper of the wind, swept through the gathering. The bee was a happy omen, relieving the solemnity of the occasion, relaxing the two main participants. And, without quite realizing it, I had relaxed, too. Though I had tried to push it to the back of my mind, the thought of sitting in a rowboat for four hours, maybe longer, would not quite go away. As the bee soared free, my spirits soared, too. I was ready for whatever might come. The minister intoned the final words, but with a twinkle in his eyes. A grinning bride and groom embraced, then walked together down the aisle and under the archway of roses, ignoring bees drawn by the seductive scent of those roses.

After the feasting Frank Savey produced his deerhide drum and told us his wife would dance. "My wife is old woman now," he said, "but she dance well . . . like when she is twelve. She dance to honor this two people here, who, like us, one day will be old, but stay together. That is good."

Sophie, brown eyes smiling, got to her feet. Around her head she slipped a band, one lone eagle feather standing upright. With one hand above her head, the other on her hip, she began her dance, a few quick stomping steps, a turn to the side, back to the front, then to the other side, a bow to Cathy, a bow to Alfred, and all accompanied by Frank's chant and the beat of his drum. When she finished she spoke in Indian to Frank.

Frank smiled. "My wife say this two people be happy now,

long time." And he added a few thoughts of his own. "Always love. Not to be ashamed. My wife and I, we love." And from the gentleness of their exchanged glances we knew that they did.

After the speech Alfred rushed up to me. "There's been a change in our plans," he whispered. "Those people that came in on the cruiser said they'd take us out to your place. They put our bags in the cruiser. No one was paying any attention to them."

"Oh!" I thought. "This is what that glimmer in Alfred's eyes was all about."

He continued gleefully, and I didn't interrupt. "Everybody's expecting us to go down to our boat at the gas dock. The cruiser's making for the seaplane float. If we head down there quickly, we can be off before anyone knows what's happened." He grinned, and I grinned, too.

We were spotted heading for the float, and as we pulled away in the cruiser I heard someone say, "Must be friends of Mrs. Flynn's. Bet they had it all planned. A dirty trick!" And it never occurred to them, I'm sure, that what they had planned was a dirty trick, too. I chuckled, pleased to have outwitted them.

There we were, three of us on a honeymoon, with two strangers not one of us had set eyes on before this day. It didn't matter. Their mood matched ours, gay and relaxed. Their participation in the honeymoon plans had added zest to a cruise through an area they had found altogether delightful. We directed them into the cove, where they pulled up alongside my skiff. The Birtles and I sat there in the skiff, watching and waving until the cruiser disappeared back up the inlet in the direction from which it had come. Only then did Alfred seize the rope and haul us in to shore.

"You kids take a walk around the beach, or wherever you wish," I said to them after we'd deposited their suitcases in an upstairs bedroom. "Stay out as long as you wish. We can have supper later. I'm sure none of us will be too hungry for a while. Really, you didn't need to have tucked in that basket of food. I ordered plenty when you told me you were coming."

"Maybe," Alfred admitted, "but you should see the way I eat. Cathy was taking no chances."

"Okay," and I laughed. "Off with you now. We'll feast when you get back."

When they came back Cathy helped me fix supper, and Alf, which suddenly seemed more appropriate than Alfred, went out to poke around in the woodshed. In a few minutes he came in, all excited.

"I didn't know you had a light plant, though I should have guessed. I've seen the house is all wired. Do you ever use it?"

"Not since Dr. Flynn died."

"Would you care if we used it tonight?"

"Not at all. There should be some gas in one of those cans in the woodshed, and there's a stand out by the north window where the generator will be far enough away from everything in case any sparks fly when you start it up."

"Great! I'll get it set up. Looks like you could use a little light in here anyway."

I smiled at his enthusiasm. It was true that we could use some light. The kitchen faced northeast, missing out on those last rays of the sun before it slipped behind Mount Eliza, so, though there was still much light outdoors, and even in the living room, the kitchen forecast the night. Night was coming earlier now, too, even outside, for with the coming of August, the long summer days when there was light in the sky until ten o'clock or later were dwindling. Still, I refrained from lighting the lamp as long as possible, for once my eyes adjusted to its light, I could see well only in that restricted area enhanced by its glow. The rest of the room would become suddenly shadowy and indistinct. It might be nice to have the old house lit up again, as Wally and I had had it on those special occasions that seemed to demand the bright lights. Certainly this night was a special occasion.

Every room in the house was bathed in a brightness I had forgotten. Alf beamed, pleased with the results. Off and on during the evening hours, however, I caught a slight frown, an uncertainty in his eyes, but he offered no explanation, and I didn't prod.

The sun smiled down on my cove that next morning, especially for my honeymooners. They strolled the beaches. They swam in the cool green waters and lay on the beach to let the sun dry and warm them, all in a sort of blissful remoteness, as if they had somehow been transported to some far world.

"It's like having your own private swimming hole," Alf exulted, in one of his more rational moments.

Later, when he was investigating the small storage rooms and the little odd cubbyholes in the old house, he came upon the 5½-horsepower outboard Wally and I had brought up when first we'd come to the cove.

"How come you have this hidden away?" he demanded, almost in disbelief, as if to say, "How could a person have such standard equipment and not use it?"

"It's not hidden," I told him, "just chucked out of the way. It's too heavy for me to lift onto the boat, and anyway," I admitted, half sheepishly, "I don't know how to run it."

He studied me a moment. I could see his thoughts. After all, I was a woman—an older woman at that.

"Tell you what," he said. "When Cathy and I go home we'll take this along. It needs some cleaning up. When I get it running good I'll bring it back and put it on your skiff and then I'll teach you how to run it. Nothing to it," he assured me.

How could I tell him I liked to row, that I actually preferred rowing, that if I had the outboard I'd still go only to those few chosen sites I rowed to? No, I couldn't tell him. He so wanted to help. At any rate, it wouldn't hurt me to learn.

Then Cathy told me: "Joe, my brother, is bringing the boat out in the morning. There's no camp at Ferrier this week, so Alf's mother and his brother want to go out and have a look around. They'll go back with Joe, and Alf and I will camp there for a few days, until Joe can come back for us."

"I'd say that sounds like fun. Ferrier Point is almost as

beautiful as the cove. Of course, I'm prejudiced, you know."

"So are we," Alf admitted, "but anyway, we want you to ride along out with us. Joe can drop you off when he takes Mum and Dave back to Esperanza."

That evening Alf made no move to start the generator. It was getting so dark inside I found myself feeling my way around.

"Alf," I said, "we're going to have to have some light in here. Do you want to start the generator?"

He hesitated a moment, then blurted out, "Do you mind if I don't? Those bright lights don't fit here. That generator fouls the air, too, takes away all the nice clean smell."

I knew then he felt about the old log house as I did, loving it as it was, without any embellishments, loving the shadowy charm that the bright lights destroyed. Then it was just another house. In the soft glow from the lamps it was beautiful and special.

Joe came early the next morning. He wanted to get through the Pacific reefs on a high tide. On a low tide the water that circulated around those reefs was so shallow a boat could get hung up on a sandbar. Then a boat had to swing far out into the Pacific, an excursion Joe felt his prairie passengers were not equal to. Down in the trough we could see no land at all; up over the swell, a quick glimpse; then down again, and always with a sideways motion. Alf's mother sat with her head bent over, her elbows resting on her knees, her hands covering her face. Dave was moaning, stretched out in the bottom of the boat.

"I thought you wanted to see Ferrier Point." Alf was totally lacking in sympathy, the motion of the sea affecting him not at all. "You're missing everything."

Dave didn't answer. He was pasty white, and his eyes rolled in their sockets. When we passed into the quiet waters of the inner harbor at Ferrier, he sat up and looked about him.

"It's okay," he said, "but you'll never get me out here again. I wouldn't go through that stretch of water again for all the horses in Alberta."

THE FLYING FLYNNS

"You're going through it again," Alf reminded him. "You've got to go back." Dave groaned.

At one time Ferrier Point had been a radar station and a long dock had extended out into the bay. Now the dock was broken and decaying. Still, on the high tide, Joe figured we could pull up to it.

"I'll try for one of those pilings," he said. "We get her snugged in, we can all go ashore."

It wasn't easy to pull up to the pilings. The sea surged in and out, threatening to bang us against a piling one moment, pulling us away the next.

"Alf," Joe directed, "get up on the bow with your rope. Dave, take the stern. Whichever end comes in closest, get a rope on something."

I stood in the stern with Dave. Joe pulled in. The bow pulled away, but the stern scraped against a piling.

"Quick, Dave," I yelled. "There's a spike. If you get your rope on it you can hold us."

He stood as if transfixed, so I jumped up on the railing and made a grab for the spike, well above my head. I had it.

"Dave! Hand me your rope."

He stood, immobile, a glassy look in his eyes, and the boat swung away. I felt my feet leave the railing, felt them dangling in space. Instinctively I had clung to that spike, a spike I wasn't sure was secure, anchored in an old piling that was rotten.

"Are you all right, Mrs. Flynn?" Alf called anxiously.

Was I all right? I looked up at the spike, wondering how long it would bear my weight, and down at the sea surging against the piling. I looked over at Dave, not quite certain how I felt about him. He was still in a trance. Suddenly, it was funny.

"Serves me right for barging in on someone else's honeymoon," I muttered to myself, but I reassured Alf. "I'm okay, for the moment anyway."

"Don't worry," he said. "Just hang on. We're coming back for you."

The weight of my body was about to pull my arm out of its socket. I considered reaching for the spike with my free hand, but hesitated, afraid that if I moved the spike would break loose from the piling. I glanced down again. A landing on the rocks at the base of the piling was guaranteed to produce bruises, if not broken bones, for the water wasn't deep enough to keep me off the rocks, and the surge of the sea would add its own measure of punishment.

Fortunately, before the spike gave way, Joe pulled in close with the boat. Alf caught me in his arms and lowered me onto the deck. Then he turned to Dave, disgust in every word he spoke.

"What's the matter with you? It isn't all that difficult to hold in a boat. It's just like tethering a horse, only with a boat you tether it at both ends."

They were both ready when Joe pulled in again, and this time the boat was tethered at both ends, with ropes around two pilings. The dock was high above the boat. We had to stand on the railing and pull ourselves up. Alf's mother refrained, insisting she could see all she wanted to from the boat, but the rest of us scrambled up, picking our way over the rotting timbers to make it to shore. We explored the camp area and then, with Cathy and Alf standing on the dock waving good-bye, we started back out the inner harbor. For me, the honeymoon was over, but it was a honeymoon I'd never forget.

Chapter 53

There was something about those latter days of August that left me feeling a bit sad. The fog drifted in more often, enclosing my world. The bright yellow leaves on my maple reminded me summer could not go on indefinitely, but what troubled me most was that August would be followed by September, and in September I would again have to return to the city. Would I be plagued by such feelings as these at the end of each summer?

As I sat on a cliff one bright morning, pondering these things, I saw a troller approaching, hugging the Nootka shoreline.

"Strange," I thought. "Today is no Harbor Day. That boat should be out fishing."

Harbor Days are those days when the wind and the sea are too rough for fishing. On such days the fishermen remain snugged to the docks at the fish camp, waiting it out or, if the weather is not too severe, risking a run to Zeballos or Tahsis for supplies the small store at camp didn't have.

I watched the troller's approach now, puzzled, until I recognized it. Alban's! My Indian neighbors took Harbor Days when a white man, insatiable in his quest for fish, would never consider it. To the Indians fishing is important, but other matters are important, too. Whatever, in their minds, is most important wins out—not necessarily fishing.

The troller turned and entered my cove. Not inclined to belittle my importance, I waved and shouted a hello, receiving a chorus in reply. Alban had brought Rose and all eight of their children. They hung over the side like monkeys, waiting for Alban to anchor and then lower the skiff. It took several trips to get them all ashore. Good thing they had come on the high tide, I reflected, so they could anchor inside the cove and not have to row too far with all those wriggling bodies. Once on shore, they tore off down the beach, in search of berries or whatever they could find.

Rose was the last to come ashore. A watchful eye had been needed on board to make certain no young daredevil hung too far over the side and kerplopped into the water. Rose was a bit heavier than when I first had met her, certainly to be expected after so many children, but her hair was still a chocolate brown, her eyes still sparkled, and in spite of a dress that fit a bit too tight, she came easily over the side of the troller and into the skiff.

"Old people tell me I am still young," she told me with a giggle.

"Old people are right," I assured her as we embraced warmly with a kiss on the cheek.

We stayed on the beach for a while, chatting over inconsequentials, watching the youngsters peg stones into the water. There was no indication that anyone was in a hurry to leave, that they might have other plans for this unscheduled Harbor Day. Alban sat on the rocks, unmoving but smiling, at peace with his world, seemingly content to just sit. I looked up at the sun, now high in the sky, then turned to Rose.

"You haven't had dinner?"

"No." She shook her head.

"You'll stay?"

"Yes, we have time. Boat's okay. Very high tide today."

"Good. It won't take me long."

She followed me up the steps and into the kitchen. While I prepared the dinner she set the long table in the living room. With so many it would be crowded, but these guests, I knew, wouldn't object to a little crowding.

Alban wandered up from the beach and sat himself in Wally's rocker. He rocked gently to and fro. It was heaven. I could see it in his face. In his house there was no rocker, yet there was no envy in his face, just pure enjoyment.

The dinner went well. Everyone was hungry and no one held back. Plates were filled and refilled. It was as it should be. There was no conversation. Eating was serious business, as well as a pleasure, and they gave it their undivided attention.

The youngsters finished and were excused. Rose and Alban and I were enjoying coffee when Rose ejected a little spark into what, on their part, had been mostly a yes and no conversation.

"Wilson's daughter is getting married," she said.

"Which daughter?" I asked.

"Mary. She is the youngest."

"Mary?" I was puzzled. "I don't seem to recall her."

"She was with her grandmother at Ahousat, but now she is home."

"Well! I bet there will be a big wedding."

"Yes. Lots of people will come. Mary will marry the son of the chief at Friendly Cove."

"How exciting!"

"Yes, but it is very sad. Wilson make no money fishing, only enough to feed his family. Mary has no wedding dress. It is not good to marry a chief's son with no wedding dress."

"That is too bad," I commiserated. "When is the wedding to be?"

"October."

"Well, maybe by then Wilson will have made a little money." I offered the only encouragement I could think of.

"Yes, maybe," she agreed doubtfully. "It is time we go now, before our boat get stuck in your cove."

I went with them down to the beach and watched as they all piled back onto the troller and cautiously made their way past my reefs. It had been wonderful, I reflected.

I was busy washing dishes when I heard the hum of another boat. At first I paid no attention. But the hum increased, seeming almost to fill the kitchen, and I had to run down to see.

By the time I reached the beach, the boat, another troller, was anchoring in the lee of my islands. A skiff, larger than Alban's, was lowered, and Paul Smith and his family, also from Nuchatlitz, rowed into the cove.

My goodness! I thought. This is certainly the day for social calls.

It was a repeat of my visit with Alban and Rose. We chatted awhile on the beach. Then I remembered my manners and asked if they'd had dinner. At Nuchatlitz one was always invited to dinner, no matter the time of day.

Julie's "No" sent me back to the kitchen. The selection in my pantry was still good. The meal was properly prepared and properly enjoyed, but at its conclusion I heard again the story of Wilson and poor Mary, with no wedding dress in which to marry the chief's son. I agreed it really was sad Wilson had made no money, and then they said it was time to go.

Again I stood on the beach, watching them leave. It had been nice, but that was enough company for one day. Keeping a hot fire going so long on a warm August day wasn't all that appealing. I had no urge to hurry back to the kitchen to wash this last batch of dishes. They could wait. I watched idly as Paul's boat rounded the curve of the island and disappeared from view, but hardly had it disappeared when another troller, appearing around the bend, brought me to startled attention.

"My God!" I exclaimed, almost in disbelief. "They're coming here, too!" I ran up to the house, flung my dishes into the dishpan, and washed them as fast as I could.

And so it went all afternoon. As soon as one boat had disappeared around the curve of the island, another appeared to take its place. My Nuchatlitz neighbors must have been waiting in line, I decided, realizing I could hardly entertain them all at once. After each visit I became a little more frantic, for no one had had dinner and the selection in my pantry had become less a matter of choice and more a matter of make-do. I was too busy preparing meals and washing dishes to wonder why they had all picked this particular day to pay me a visit.

Not one of them, however, forgot to relate the story of poor Wilson and poor Mary, and I must confess that with each retelling I became less and less inclined to commiserate.

By 6:30 that evening, when the latest troller left, I had reached a state of nervous exhaustion. They all had such large families. Children were wonderful, I conceded, but not when you had to feed them all in one day. Surely now no more boats would come. I must have fed everyone in Nuchatlitz. Still, I watched warily as this last troller rounded the curve. Ah! No troller appeared to take its place. I stood for a moment, my eyes fixed, almost doubting my good fortune. Then I turned and slowly climbed the steps to clear away that last batch of dishes.

I had barely finished when I heard the roar of an outboard. The roar came into the cove and I had to go down. A young man was already anchoring the boat to one of the boulders on the beach. He was a handsome fellow, coal-black hair, dark brown eyes, and a flashing smile that seemed to say, "I'm a friend." His companion, a young girl, sat quietly in the boat, her eyes downcast. Neither spoke a word, and I couldn't recall having seen either before. At least, I thought, they will have had dinner. It was past seven o'clock, but they hadn't eaten, they said.

"It's late. You must be awfully hungry. Come on up to the house and we'll see what we can do about it."

Again that flashing smile from the youth. "She will go with you," he said, nodding toward the girl. "If you give me a hammer and some nails, I will find something to fix."

It was uncomfortably quiet in the kitchen as, once more, I prepared dinner. My guest sat like a statue, staring at the floor. I could draw from her not even a yes or a no, and after a while, tired of supplying answers to my own questions, I gave up, wishing Mama were here with her unending supply of jokes, wishing I had been likewise gifted. It was with a real sense of relief that I called the young man to dinner. At least he could smile. And in his presence the girl relaxed, to a degree. I asked what he'd found to fix, and he told me he'd found an old boardwalk back in the bush around the beach and had nailed down boards that had worked free of their underpinnings.

And all the while he talked I thought to myself, "Who are they?" And then I thought, "Well, why don't you ask?" Indian people never ask outright. In spite of using very few words, they always managed to work around to what they wanted.

"I've been trying to place you," I said, "but I just can't recall having seen either of you before. You are from Nuchat-litz?"

He nodded. "She is."

And suddenly a great light dawned. I turned to the girl. "Are you Mary?" I asked.

She nodded.

"Do you want me to buy you a wedding dress?"

She nodded again, and from the young man—the groom, of course—came that buoyant smile.

"Okay," I said. "When I leave to go back to Seattle I'll stop off in Vancouver and buy you a wedding dress. I wish I could deliver it myself, but I'll mail it and you'll get it in plenty of time for the wedding. Stand up. Let's see how near of a size we are."

I would have liked to have attended that wedding, but a trip back out, with the additional expense of a wedding gown, was more than my limited budget could stand. Their reasoning, however, was obvious now. Anyone who had owned a plane had to be rich. It was not necessarily so. Whatever, the shy, sweet smile with which Mary rewarded my offer rendered the cost of the garment immaterial.

Pretty clever neighbors I had, I reflected after my two young guests had departed. Never would they have asked outright. The offer had to come from me. Even with all the wearing down, the plan had almost failed. It had taken Mary herself, a very reluctant Mary, to break through my armor of indifference. Then I grinned. It was not every day one got to feed an entire village.

Chapter 54

With the wind whistling through the trees and the rain pattering on the roof, the evocative serenade of bush country, it seemed I had never been away. I'd gone to Vancouver in September. I'd bought that wedding dress, trying on several before I found just the right one—white, of course, and ankle length, so it wouldn't get soiled as Mary walked over the humpy earth to the church. I'd ignored the furtive smirks of the clerks. A woman my age in a wedding gown! The long winter months also had been pleasant, but they blurred now into nothingness. This was the real world. This was the real me, this scroungy waif who ran bare-legged in the rain, who cut wood to keep warm, ignoring the ping of raindrops in those pans on the floor. Ah! This was the good life.

A bang on the door brought me out of my chair. Father Larkin's ample form appeared in the door window, and I waved him in.

I greeted him. "What are you doing out in weather like this?"

He grinned down at me. "In weather like this people still need a priest." Then the joking mood vanished into a frown. "This is ridiculous!" he sputtered.

"I don't get you," I said, irritation in my voice.

"All these damn pans sitting around the room!"

"And what would you suggest?" I asked sweetly.

"I'd suggest you get your roof reshingled."

"That's easier said than done."

"Maybe so; maybe not. If you can find a place to hang this jacket where it won't get wet, we'll see if we can think this thing out."

I took the jacket, refraining from observing aloud that it was already wet. Father Larkin, I knew from times past, had a quick tongue and was an incorrigible tease, but he also had a way of working things out.

"How about lunch while we're deciding what to do about my leaky roof?" I suggested.

"Good idea, only maybe you'd better make it dinner. Weather like this stirs up a man's appetite. Anyway, I hear tell you're quite good at cooking up dinners."

I wrinkled my nose at him, choosing to ignore as best I could his reference to Mary's dilemma and my density in recognizing a solution. "Dinner will take longer," I cautioned him.

"So? Who said anything about being in a hurry?"

"Nobody," I admitted, "but you always are."

"Well, let's just say that today I'm not, and now that we've got that settled, let's get back to our original concern."

"It's going to have to stay a concern, Father. I don't have the money."

He shrugged it off. "Who has? That's no problem. Must be something around here you can sell. I'll have a look around while you stir up whatever you're stirring up there."

I went ahead with my dinner preparations, and he wandered into the living room. I could hear him poking around, all the while whistling some tune I didn't recognize.

"Say!" he called out after a bit. "Darn fine-looking adding machine you've got here. Do you ever use it?" he asked, coming to stand in the doorway.

"Not anymore. All the figuring I need to do up here I can do in my head."

"Well then, why keep it around?"

"Oh, I don't know. Haven't known what to do with it, I guess."

"Sell it! That'll buy your shingles. An adding machine is just what Wes needs in that store at Queens Cove."

"He might not think so."

"I'll take it over and tell him. In exchange for the adding machine he can order you some shingles from Port Alberni and have them delivered to Queens Cove on the *Packer* its next trip up."

"Even if he agrees," I hedged, "how would I ever get all those shingles over here?"

"Wilson! He can get one of the boys to help him. He owes you a favor."

"I doubt he'll agree with that."

"He will after I've talked with him."

"Honestly, Father," I protested, "you can't go around telling everybody what they want to do."

"I can't?" He grinned, a big grin, spreading all over his face and into his eyes.

I took in the grin and the size of him, and I laughed. "I guess you can," I admitted. "But I sure don't know anything about shingling a roof."

"Women!" he snorted. "They can think up excuses faster than a man can breathe. Even God must find them trying at times. Have faith, woman. The Lord will provide. And isn't that dinner about ready? My stomach's about to flip just smelling it. A man can't stand around all day. I got places to go."

In a hurry again, but despite his seeming urgency, he ate a leisurely dinner, and in the process made a suggestion that pleased me. How would I like it if he stopped in someday and took me along to Nuchatlitz? I could attend Mass, visit around for a while, and probably get invited to dinner. When he left he took my adding machine with him, covered with an old rain jacket to protect it from the weather. I promptly forgot all about it.

I did not, however, forget about that promised trip to

Nuchatlitz. When he stopped in again, about a week later, I was raring to go.

"Should I wear a dress, Father?" I asked.

"Would be nice, if you have one. You'll feel more comfortable. They all put on their best to come to Mass."

I wouldn't feel altogether comfortable anyway, I was to discover. I went directly to Rose's house and visited with her while she got her family ready. Then, when Father rang the church bell, we strolled the hundred yards to the church, sidestepping the cow chips, some quite fresh, that were strewn in our path.

We joined others approaching the small white frame building, churchly in appearance, with a steeple and a bell tower. I nodded to my friends and with them filed into the church, taking my place with Rose and her family. I was glad I'd worn a dress. Father Larkin appeared from some back room and disappeared into the confessional, a boxlike affair with a curtain across the front to insure a degree of privacy. Minutes passed. Nobody had moved. I darted a furtive glance around. Everyone was staring straight ahead, passive, expressionless.

What were they waiting for? I wondered. It must be awfully hot in that box. Father would get discouraged and come out if somebody didn't go in there pretty darn quick. I knew his impatience. I glanced around again. Everyone seemed glued to their seats. Then the thought struck me. Could they be waiting for me? I was a guest. Common courtesy gave me the option of being first. Option? No choice at all, really, and certainly something I wasn't prepared for. Having lived most of my life as a Protestant, I'd found it hard, since becoming a Catholic, to see any real need to confess my sins to another human.

If I refused to go in, maybe someone else would go. Still, no one moved, nor did Father come out. He could suffocate in there. Maybe he already had. I should go see. I slid forward on the bench. Rose smiled encouragement. I got up, stumbling over the feet of the youngster who sat beside me, and made my way slowly down the aisle.

As I approached the confessional I recalled what Father Noonan had told me of an Indian child making her first confession at Christie. She had knelt there in the dark for some time, not saying a word.

Thinking to help her, Father Noonan had whispered, "Are you scared?"

"No," she'd whispered back. "Are you?"

At the time it had seemed funny. Now it didn't seem so funny. For me there was no shield of anonymity. It made no difference that in that box Father couldn't see me. Mine was the only non-Indian voice in the entire congregation. Gathering up what courage I could, I pushed the curtain aside and stepped into the darkness. I knelt, hesitated, then blurted out, "You already know everything I've done. For whatever I've done wrong, I'm sorry."

He mumbled the usual words and then said, "For your pennance, say one Hail Mary."

"Is that all?" I exclaimed.

"I think that will take care of it."

Did I detect a hint of laughter in his voice? It didn't matter. I got to my feet and pushed through the curtain, glad to have escaped from that hot little box. Rose passed me in the aisle, and as I knelt, obediently, to recite my Hail Mary, I was conscious of others lining up to make their confessions. It had taken me long enough to get things moving. I wondered if Father Larkin would bother to bring me again.

He did, and I came to look forward to those trips to Nuchatlitz, accepting their irregularity. Mass was not held specifically on Sundays. Distances between villages was great, thirty miles or more. Weather was always a factor. Mass was when Father got there. It could be a week and a half, two weeks, even three. Time between was immaterial. It mattered only that he came. I treasured my visits with each family, going from house to house, and especially I delighted in the meal Rose prepared after every service. It was pleasant eating with friends.

Father Larkin wasn't my only visitor, however. Cathy and

Alf came in one day, bringing my outboard. We'd decided, last August, that he might as well keep it all winter, since I wouldn't be using it anyway. Now he attached it to my skiff and started it up. It purred, smooth as honey.

"Beautiful!" he crowed. "Come on, get in. I'll show you how to run it."

I wasn't the best pupil around, but Alf was patient, and after a time I began to feel comfortable with that lever in my hand, turning the skiff to the right or the left, whatever my fancy. It gave me a sweet feeling of power—man over machine—but it didn't extend my horizons. I took it only to those places I'd rowed, but because I could go faster, I went more often. Rowing, however, remained my first love, and I spent hours testing my strength against the roll of the sea.

Cathy and Al weren't free to come out too often. Cathy worked as a nurse's aide at the hospital. Alf was in charge of boat repairs and general maintenance, and there were always things at Esperanza that needed fixing, but when they did come it was like a fresh breeze blowing in off the salt. Their youth, their vigor, their willingness to tackle jobs that were too difficult for me, or just plain too boring, sparked my day.

Around an old log house Alf could always find something needing repair, and there was generally a log to saw into rolls, one I'd hauled in with a peevee as it floated by my beach. With a nail bent over a rope in one end of the log, I'd tie it to a cedar branch, where it would ride the tides until Alf appeared to take over. Cathy found work to do, too, washing those windows I'd neglected, helping me chop and pack wood. I sometimes protested that they did too much, but they brushed my objections aside.

"Coming out here is the most fun we have," Alf told me. "It isn't something we have to do. It's something we want to do. And we have the boat trip coming and going."

"Yes," Cathy interrupted him, laughing, "and there's no place he'd rather be than in that boat. Sometimes I think he loves that boat more than me."

Alf grinned. "Let's say it's equal. Actually, what we both love is this old house and your cove."

One evening when the tide was high, a troller chugged into the cove. Wilson. I recognized the boat. Then I recognized him, his head poking through the side window of the troller, and, yes, Pat, standing on the deck beside a pile of . . . of shingles?

Wilson's shout confirmed my suspicion. "We bring your shingles. Where you want them?"

Where did I want them? It had been over six weeks since Father Larkin had walked off with my adding machine. I hadn't thought of it again, or of the shingles, either. To me they represented just one more problem, a problem I doubted could be as easily solved as he had intimated.

"I don't know, Wilson," I called back. "Stack them on the first level, I guess. At least the tide won't get them there."

Wilson anchored the troller, and Pat shoved the skiff into the water. Back and forth, between the troller and the shore, and the stack of shingles on that first level seemed to grow out of all proportions. Sure, my kitchen was big, twenty-four by fourteen feet, according to Father Larkin's estimate.

"Could one fair-to-middling adding machine buy all those shingles?"

I was allowed to dwell on this troubling supposition unin- terrupted. There was no small talk between Pat and Wilson, or with me, as they worked. Small talk is an idiosyncrasy of the white man.

"All done," Wilson announced at last, wiping his forehead with the back of his hand. "Father want them shingles some- place else, he can move them hisself." But he was grinning, and I knew he wasn't angry he'd been imposed upon. Pat was grinning, too.

"See you sometime," Wilson continued, "when you have no more shingles to move."

And I grinned as I waved. "See you, Pat, Wilson!" Certainly I wouldn't want the Lord to provide more than was my due.

In the days that followed, however, and in spite of the

rich cedar smell they shed, those shingles were more of a source of annoyance than of pleasure. I couldn't go up or down the steps without going around them. They pricked at my conscience, a constant reminder of my inadequacies. Maybe God intended I should shingle the roof myself. If I meant to stay up here, I shouldn't hesitate to tackle the job. I scolded and harangued, seeking to prod my rebellious nature into action. I went so far as to try to lift one of the bundles, and found that I couldn't. To get those shingles up the steps to the house, I would have to break open the bundles and carry the shingles up a few at a time. The task assumed herculean proportions.

"Drat!" I exploded, kicking at one of the bundles, and I went for a walk, a long, long walk, as far up the beach as I dared, hoping to rid myself of the thought of those shingles. It didn't help much, because when I got back the shingles were still there. Minniebelle strutted ahead of me down the path, a picture of lofty unconcern. She flew to a branch in the plum tree, where she cocked her head to the side, regarding me disapprovingly.

"What's the matter with you?" I think she said. "It's a beautiful world. Shame on you, going around with that scowl on your face, kicking at things. You're not very good company."

And I realized she was right. Why, the squirrels and the mink and even the overbearing crows had darted out of my way as I'd scuffed along, kicking at stones and pieces of drift.

"I'm sorry, Minniebelle," I said, and I felt better. Father Larkin had said the Lord would provide, but he hadn't said when. I'd have to learn to be patient.

I talked to my squirrels and told them it was okay. "Sit there and enjoy whatever that is you're eating. You don't have to run away from me."

I found Jasper, my mink, sniffing among the bundles. "Smells super, doesn't it?" And I'm sure he agreed.

I walked on the beach and I picked up my feet, walking lightly, whistling as I went. The crows merely stepped to the side, ignoring me as before. Life had settled back into its normal pattern.

And then one day I spotted a boat coming my way and soon recognized it as Alf's. As he leaped from the boat to the shore, his head was up, his nostrils tightening as he sniffed the air.

"Cedar!" he exclaimed. "Man, does that smell good. What have you got?"

"Shingles," I replied. "Come and see."

Cathy leaped ashore, too, and after the anchor rope was secured around a boulder, they followed me up to the first level.

"Wow! Beautiful!" Alf's eyes were wide with wonder. "Where did you get them?"

"Father Larkin had them sent up to Queens Cove on the *Packer*. He said my kitchen roof was a disgrace."

Alf's laughter was spontaneous. "I guess it is, all right. Hey!" he exclaimed as a thought struck him. "Could Cathy and I shingle your roof? That would be great fun."

His enthusiasm was contagious, and Cathy and I were soon working right alongside him. He broke the bundles apart so we could help carry the shingles up to the house. Fleetingly, I regretted that someone had wanted the little winch Wally had installed at the top of the embankment. He had laid wooden rails from the first level and had rigged up a cart with old wheels he'd found lying around. We'd used the winch and the cart for everything—groceries for our larder, wood for the stove, furniture for the house. Now the cart sat forlornly at the bottom, unable to go anywhere. I'd tried to ignore it, determined the loss would not upset me, knowing it would have to have been taken by a stranger, knowing none of my friends and neighbors would do anything to make it harder for me to live here. I'd pretty well succeeded, but for the moment now I resented that stranger. However, with Alf and Cathy laughing and joking as they worked along with me, it became, as Alf had said, great fun.

Cathy and Alf swept the roof clean, making sure no bits of dry moss clung to the sun-baked shingles. The new shingles went on over the old, with Cathy handing out the shingles and Alf nailing them in place.

One thing I knew for certain. With a new roof on the old house, I wouldn't be in any great hurry to renege on my resolve to live at the cove. For as many years as I chose to live here, I would be snug and warm in my old log house.